Counsels on the Dangers of Prescription Drugs

Including Simple Home Remedies for Replacing Many Medications

A Compilation from the Writings of

Ellen G. White

"After seeing so much harm done by the administering of drugs, I cannot use them, and cannot testify in their favor. I must be true to the light given me by the Lord."

Letter 82, 1897

Printed in the USA

Compiled and published by:

Veggies Health Food Center
1202 Brookview Drive
Ardmore, Oklahoma 73401

(580) 226-2424

Table of Contents

Counsels on the Dangers of Prescription Drugs

Preface

A "silent epidemic," side effects from the use of prescription drugs rank third in the leading causes of death in the United States today, right behind heart disease and cancer (as stated by T. Colin Campbell in his new book, *Whole*).

What we are not talking about here are illegal drugs that our country spends millions of dollars "warring" against. Rather, it is the pharmaceutical drugs, appropriately prescribed (according to modern medicine), that are resulting in over a hundred thousand deaths per year.

In light of this disturbing trend, the words penned in this easy-to-read book have never been more relevant than they are today. Though written more than a century ago, and at times referring to outdated pharmaceutical drugs, they are exactly what we need. Unfortunately, prescription drugs are just as poisonous today as they were back then. If this little book were heeded, I believe there would be far fewer people suffering and dying today from the side effects of commonly prescribed medications.

My prayer is that this compilation will open your eyes, not only to how detrimental the use of pharmaceutical drugs can be, but also to the wonderful benefits of simple natural remedies. *We wish above all things that you will prosper and be in health.*

Mary Bernt

Dangers of Reliance on Drugs

A Shortcut that Fetters Nature

The human family has brought upon themselves diseases of various forms by their own wrong habits. They have not studied how to live healthfully, and their transgression of the laws of their being has produced a deplorable state of things. The people have seldom accredited their sufferings to the true cause—their own wrong course of action. They have indulged an intemperance in eating, and made a god of their appetite. In all their habits they have manifested a recklessness in regard to health and life; and when, as the result, sickness has come upon them they have made themselves believe that God was the author of it, when their own wrong course of action has brought the sure result. When in distress they send for the doctor, and trust their bodies in his hands, expecting that he will make them well. He deals out to them drugs, the nature of which they know nothing, and in their blind confidence they swallow anything that the doctor may choose to give. Thus powerful poisons are often administered which fetter nature in all her friendly efforts to recover the abuse the system has suffered, and the patient is hurried out of this life.

How to Live, page 49

Wonderful Cures that Kill

The endless variety of medicines in the market, the numerous advertisements of new drugs and mixtures, all of which, as they say, do wonderful cures, kill hundreds where they benefit one. Those who are sick are not patient. They will take the various medicines, some of which are very powerful, although they know nothing of the nature of the mixtures. All the medicines they take only make their recovery more hopeless. Yet they keep dosing, and continue to grow weaker, until they die. Some will have medicine at all events. Then let them take these hurtful mixtures and the various deadly poisons upon their own responsibility. God's servants should not administer medicines which they know will leave behind injurious effects upon the system, even if they do relieve present suffering.

Every poisonous preparation in the vegetable and mineral kingdoms, taken into the system, will leave its wretched influence, affecting the liver and lungs, and deranging the system generally. Nor does the evil end here. Diseased, feeble infants are brought into the world to share this misery, transmitted to them from their parents.

Spiritual Gifts, Vol. IV, pages 139-140

Many, instead of seeking to remove the poisonous matter from the system, take a more deadly poison into the system to remove a poison already there.

Healthful Living, page 243

Drugs Injure the System

Every pernicious drug placed in the human stomach, whether by prescription of physicians or by man himself, doing violence to the human organism, injures the whole machinery. Every intemperate indulgence of lustful appetite is at war with natural instinct and the healthful condition of every nerve and muscle and organ of the wonderful human machinery which through the Creator's power possesses organic life.

Nature would do her work wisely and well if the human agent would, in his treatment of the body, cooperate with the divine purpose. But how Satan and his whole confederacy rejoice to see how easily his powers of deception and art can persuade men to form an appetite for most unpleasant stimulants and narcotics. And then when nature has been overborne, enfeebled in all her working force, there is the drug medication to come from the physicians, to kill the remaining vital force and leave men miserable wrecks of suffering, of imbecility, of insanity, and of loathsome disease. God is hidden from the human observation by the hellish shadow of Satan.

Selected Messages Book 2, pages 280-281

A practice that is laying the foundation of a vast amount of disease and of even more serious evils, is the free use of poisonous drugs. When attacked by disease, many will not take the trouble to search out the cause of their illness. Their chief anxiety is to rid themselves of pain and inconvenience. So they resort to patent nostrums, of whose real properties they know little, or they apply to a physician for some remedy to counteract the result of their misdoing, but with no thought of making a change in their unhealthful habits. If immediate benefit is not realized, another medicine is tried, and then another. Thus the evil continues.

Ministry of Healing, page 126

Many act as if health and disease were things entirely independent of their conduct, and entirely outside their control. They do not reason from cause to effect, and submit to feebleness and disease as a necessity. Violent attacks of sickness they believe to be special dispensations of Providence, or the result of some overruling, mastering power; and they resort to drugs as a cure for the evil. But the drugs taken to cure the disease weaken the system.

Medical Ministry, pages 296-297

Drugs given to stupefy, whatever they may be, derange the nervous system.

How to Live, No. 3, page 57

Poison to the Blood

Brother B seeks to have his wife believe as he believes, and he would have her think that all he does is right and that he knows more than any of the ministers and is wise above all men. I was shown that in his boasted wisdom he is dealing with the bodies of his children as he is with the soul of his wife. He has been following a course according to his own wisdom, which is ruining the health of his child. He flatters himself that the poison which he has introduced into her system keeps her alive. What a mistake! He should reason how much better she might have been had he let her alone and not abused nature. This child can never have a sound constitution, for her bones and the current of blood in her veins have been poisoned. The shattered constitutions of his children and their aches and distressing pains will cry out against his boasted wisdom, which is folly.

Testimonies, Vol. 3, page 454

When the abuse of health is carried so far that sickness results, the sufferer can often do for himself what no one else can do for him. The first thing to be done is to ascertain the true character of the sickness, and then go to work intelligently to remove the cause. If the harmonious working of the system has become unbalanced by overwork, overeating, or other irregularities, do not endeavor to adjust the difficulties by adding a burden of poisonous medicines.

Ministry of Healing, page 235

In our sanitariums, we advocate the use of simple remedies. We discourage the use of drugs, for they poison the current of the blood. In these institutions sensible instruction should be given how to eat, how to drink, how to dress, and how to live so that the health may be preserved.

Counsels on Diet and Foods, page 303

Do not endeavor to adjust the difficulties by adding a burden of poisonous medicines.

The Ministry of Healing, pages 235

Drugs always have a tendency to break down and destroy vital forces.

Medical Ministry, page 223

A Curse to the Human Race

If those who take these drugs were alone the sufferers, then the evil would not be as great. But parents not only sin against themselves in swallowing drug-poisons, but they sin against their children. The vitiated state of their blood, the poison distributed throughout the system, the broken constitution, and various drug-diseases, as the result of drug-poisons, are transmitted to their offspring, and left them as a wretched inheritance, which is another great cause of the degeneracy of the race.

How to Live, page 50

Physicians, by administering their drug-poisons, have done very much to increase the depreciation of the race, physically, mentally, and morally. Everywhere you may go you will see deformity, disease and imbecility, which in very many cases can be traced directly back to the drug-poisons, administered by the hand of a doctor, as a remedy for some of life's ills. The so-called remedy has fearfully proved itself to the patient, by stern suffering experience, to be far worse than the disease for which the drug was taken. All who possess common capabilities should understand the wants of their own system. The philosophy of health should compose one of the important studies for our children. It is all-important that the human organism be understood, and then intelligent men and women can be their own physicians. If the people would reason from cause to effect, and would follow the light which shines upon them, they would pursue a course which would insure health, and mortality would be far less. But the people are too willing to remain in inexcusable ignorance, and trust their bodies to the doctors, instead of having any special responsibility in the matter themselves.

Selected Messages Book 2, pages 442-443

A Leading Cause of Death

I was shown that more deaths have been caused by drug-taking than from all other causes combined. If there was in the land one physician in the place of thousands, a vast amount of premature mortality would be prevented. Multitudes of physicians, and multitudes of drugs, have cursed the inhabitants of the earth, and have carried thousands and tens of thousands to untimely graves.

Indulging in eating too frequently, and in too large quantities, over-taxes the digestive organs, and produces a feverish state of the system. The blood becomes impure, and then diseases of various kinds occur. A physician is sent for, who prescribes some drug which gives present relief, but which does not cure the disease. It may change the form of disease, but the real evil is increased tenfold. Nature was doing her best to rid the system of an accumulation of impurities, and could she have been left to herself, aided by the common blessings of Heaven, such as pure air and pure water, a speedy and safe cure would have been effected.

The sufferers in such cases can do for themselves that which others cannot do as well for them. They should commence to relieve nature of the load they have forced upon her. They should remove the cause. Fast a short time, and give the stomach chance for rest. Reduce the feverish state of the system by a careful and understanding application of water. These efforts will help nature in her struggles to free the system of impurities. But generally the persons who suffer pain become impatient. They are not willing to use self-denial, and suffer a little from hunger. Neither are they willing to wait the slow process of nature to build up the overtaxed energies of the system. But they are determined to obtain relief at once, and take powerful drugs, prescribed by physicians. Nature was doing her work well, and would have triumphed, but while accomplishing her task, a foreign substance of a poisonous nature was introduced. What a mistake! Abused nature has now two evils to war against instead of one. She leaves the work in which she was engaged, and resolutely takes hold to expel the intruder newly introduced into the system. Nature feels this double draft upon her resources, and she becomes enfeebled.

Spiritual Gifts, Vol. IV, pages 133-134

More deaths have been caused by drug-taking than from all other causes combined.

Selected Messages Book 2, pages 450

There is a disposition with many parents, to keep up a perpetual dosing of their children with medicines. They will always have a supply on hand, and when any slight indisposition is manifested, caused by overeating or exhaustion, the medicine is poured down their throats; and if that does not satisfy them, they send for the doctor. If he is an honest physician, and declines to give the child medicine because he is wise enough to know it will be for its hurt, the parents are offended and think the physician inefficient, and send for another, who is less conscientious, and who will give medicine to satisfy the parents, who were blinded by ignorance in regard to the real condition and need of their child. And not infrequently parents are so anxious to do all they can to save their child, that they change physicians, having two or three to attend the same

13

case. The child is drugged to death, and the parents console themselves that they have done all they could, and wonder why it must die when they did so much to save it. Upon the gravestone of that child should be written, Died, of Drug Medication.

Health Reformer
September 1866

Health Lost Through Drugs

Multitudes remain in inexcusable ignorance in regard to the laws of their being. They are wondering why our race is so feeble, and why so many die prematurely. Is there not a cause? Physicians who profess to understand the human organism, prescribe for their patients, and even for their own dear children, and their companions, slow poisons to break up disease, or to cure slight indisposition. Surely, they cannot realize the evil of these things as they were presented before me, or they could not do thus. The effects of the poison may not be immediately perceived, but it is doing its work surely in the system, undermining the constitution, and crippling nature in her efforts. They are seeking to correct an evil, but produce a far greater one, which is often incurable.

Those who are thus dealt with are constantly sick, and constantly dosing. And yet, if you listen to their conversation, you will often hear them praising the drugs they have been using, and recommending their use to others, because they have been benefited by their use. It would seem that to such as can reason from cause to effect, the sallow countenance, the continual complaints of ailments and general prostration of those who claim to be benefited, would be sufficient proofs of the health-destroying influence of drugs. And yet many are so blinded they do not see that all the drugs they have taken have not cured them, but made them worse. The drug invalid numbers one in the world, but is generally peevish, irritable, always sick, lingering out a miserable existence, and seems to live only to call into constant exercise the patience of others. Poisonous drugs have not killed them outright, for nature is loath to give up her hold on life. She is unwilling to cease her struggles. Yet these drug-takers are never well. They are always taking cold, which causes extreme suffering, because of the poison all through their system.

Spiritual Gifts, Vol. IV, pages 137-138

By the use of poisonous drugs, many bring upon themselves lifelong illness, and many lives are lost that might be saved by the use of natural methods of healing. The poisons contained in many so-called remedies create habits and appetites that mean ruin to both soul and body. Many of the popular nostrums called patent medicines, and even some of the drugs dispensed by physicians, act a part in laying the foundation of the liquor habit, the opium habit, the morphine habit, that are so terrible a curse to society.

Ministry of Healing, pages 126-127

Drugs Never Cure Disease

Use nature's remedies—water, sunshine, and fresh air. Do not use drugs. Drugs never heal; they only change the features of the disease.

The Paulson Collection of Ellen G. White Letters. page 17

People need to be taught that drugs do not cure disease. It is true that they sometimes afford present relief, and the patient appears to recover as the result of their use; this is because nature has sufficient vital force to expel the poison and to correct the conditions that caused the disease. Health is recovered in spite of the drug. But in most cases the drug only changes the form and location of the disease. Often the effect of the poison seems to be overcome for a time, but the results remain in the system and work great harm at some later period.

Ministry of Healing, page 126

Drugs never cure disease. They only change the form and location. Nature alone is the effectual restorer, and how much better could she perform her task if left to herself. But this privilege is seldom allowed her. If crippled nature bears up under the load, and finally accomplishes in a great measure her double task, and the patient lives, the credit is given to the physician. But if nature fails in her effort to expel the poison from the system, and the patient dies, it is called a wonderful dispensation of Providence. If the patient had taken a course to relieve overburdened nature in season, and understandingly used pure soft water, this dispensation of drug mortality might have been wholly averted. The use of water can accomplish but little, if the patient does not feel the necessity of also strictly attending to his diet.

Many are living in violation of the laws of health, and are ignorant of the relation their habits of eating, drinking, and working sustain to their health. They will not arouse to their true condition until nature protests against the abuses she is suffering, by aches and pains in the system. If, even then, the sufferers would only commence the work right, and would resort to the simple means they have neglected—the use of water and proper diet, nature would have just the help she requires, and which she ought to have had long before. If this course is pursued, the patient will generally recover, without being debilitated.

When drugs are introduced into the system, for a time they may seem to have a beneficial effect. A change may take place, but the disease is not cured. It will manifest itself in some other form. In nature's efforts to expel the drug from the system, intense suffering is sometimes caused the patient. And the disease, which the drug was given to cure, may disappear, but only to re-appear in a new form, such as skin diseases, ulcers, painful diseased joints, and sometimes in a more dangerous and deadly form. The liver, heart and brain are frequently affected by drugs, and often all these organs are burdened with disease, and the unfortunate subjects, if they live, are invalids for life, wearily dragging out a miserable existence. Oh, how much that poisonous drug cost! If it did not cost the life, it cost quite too much. Nature has been crippled in all her efforts. The whole machinery is out of order, and at a future period in life, when these fine works which have been injured, are to be relied upon to act a more important part in union with all the fine works of nature's machinery, they cannot readily and strongly perform their labor, and the whole system feels the lack. These organs, which should be in a healthy condition, are enfeebled, the blood becomes impure. Nature keeps struggling, and the patient suffers with different ailments, until there is a sudden breaking down in her efforts, and death follows. There are more who die from the use of drugs, than all who could have died of disease had nature been left to do her own work.

Very many lives have been sacrificed by physicians' administering drugs for unknown diseases. They have no real knowledge of the exact disease which afflicts the patient. But physicians are expected to know in a moment what to do, and unless they act at once, as though they understood the disease perfectly, they are considered by impatient friends, and by the sick, as incompetent physicians. Therefore to gratify erroneous opinions of the sick and their friends, medicine must be administered, experiments and tests tried to cure the patient of the disease of which they have no real knowledge. Nature is loaded with poisonous drugs which she cannot expel from the system. The physicians themselves are often convinced that they have used powerful medicines for a disease which did not exist, and death was the consequence.

Spiritual Gifts, Vol. IV, pages 134-136

Impatience is Part of the Problem

Physicians are censurable, but they are not the only ones at fault. The sick themselves, if they would be patient, diet and suffer a little, and give nature time to rally, would recover much sooner without the use of any medicine. NATURE ALONE POSSESSES CURATIVE POWERS. Medicines have no power to cure, but will most generally hinder nature in her efforts. She after all must do the work of restoring. The sick are in a hurry to get well, and the friends of the sick are impatient. They will have medicine, and if they do not feel that powerful influence upon their systems, their erroneous views lead them to think they should feel, they impatiently change for another physician. The change often increases the evil. They go through a course of medicine equally as dangerous as the first, and more fatal, because the two treatments do not agree, and the system is poisoned beyond remedy.

Spiritual Gifts, Vol. IV, ppage 136

The sick are in a hurry to get well, and the friends of the sick are impatient. They will have medicine, and if they do not feel that powerful influence upon their systems their erroneous views lead them to think they should feel, they impatiently change for another physician. The change often increases the evil. They go through a course of medicine equally as dangerous as the first.

How to Live, No. 3, page 62

Ignorance is Not an Excuse

Our institutions are established that the sick may be treated by hygienic methods, discarding almost entirely the use of drugs...There is a terrible account to be rendered to God by men who have so little regard for human life as to treat the body so ruthlessly in dealing out their drugs...We are not excusable if through ignorance we destroy God's building by taking into our stomachs poisonous drugs under a variety of names we do not understand. It is our duty to refuse all such prescriptions.

Healthful Living, page 246

Stories of Sickness and Healing

This story of prescription drug use, as written by Ellen White, represents only one of many such incidents which are happening with all too much frequency. The remaining stories in this chapter, which were interwoven together when written, have been regrouped so that the reader can read one story at a time.

A Young Mother Laid in the Grave

The mother who has been but slightly indisposed, and who might have recovered by abstinence from food for a short period, and a cessation from labor, having quiet and rest, has, instead of doing this, sent for a physician. And he who should be prepared to understandingly give a few simple directions, and restrictions in diet, and place her upon the right track, is either too ignorant to do this, or too anxious to obtain a fee.

He makes the case a grave one, and administers his poisons, which, if he were sick, he would not venture to take himself. The patient grows worse, and poisonous drugs are more freely administered, until nature is overpowered in her efforts, and gives up the conflict, and the mother dies. She was drugged to death. Her system was poisoned beyond remedy. She was murdered. Neighbors and relatives marvel at the wonderful dealings of providence in thus removing a mother in the midst of her usefulness, at the period when her children need her care so much. They wrong our good and wise heavenly Father when they cast back upon him this weight of human woe.

Heaven wished that mother to live, and her untimely death dishonored God. The mother's wrong habits, and her inattention to the laws of her being, made her sick. And the doctor's fashionable poisons, introduced into the system, closed the period of her existence, and left a helpless, stricken, motherless flock.

The above is not always the result which follows the doctor's drugging. Sick people who take these drug-poisons do appear to get well. With some, there is sufficient life-force for nature to draw upon, to so far expel the poison from the system that the sick, having a period of rest, recover. But no credit should be allowed the drugs taken, for they only hindered nature in her efforts. ALL THE CREDIT SHOULD BE ASCRIBED TO NATURE'S RESTORATIVE POWERS.

Although the patient may recover, yet the powerful effort nature was required to make to induce action to overcome the poison, injured the constitution, and shortened the life of the patient. There are many who do not die under the influence of drugs, but there are very many who are left useless wrecks, hopeless, gloomy, and miserable sufferers, a burden to themselves and to society.

Selected Messages Book 2, pages 441-442

The Case of One Father and Daughter

Ellen White tells the touching story of one father and daughter who had already sustained great loss:

The daughter was sick, and the father was much troubled on her account, and summoned a physician. As the father conducted him into the sick room, he manifested a painful anxiety. The physician examined the patient, and said but little. They both left the sick room. The father informed the physician that he had buried the mother, a son and daughter, and this daughter was all that was left to him of his family. He anxiously inquired of the physician if he thought his daughter's case hopeless.

The physician then inquired in regard to the nature and length of the sickness of those who had died. The father mournfully related the painful facts connected with the illness of his loved ones.

My son was first attacked with a fever. I called a physician. He said that he could administer medicine which would soon break the fever. He gave him powerful medicine, but was disappointed in its effects. The fever was reduced, but my son grew dangerously sick. The same medicine was again given him, without producing any change for the better. The physician then resorted to still more powerful medicines, but my son obtained no relief. The fever left him, but he did not rally. He sank rapidly and died.

The death of my son so sudden and unexpected was a great grief to us all, but especially to his mother. Her watching and anxiety in his sickness, and her grief occasioned by his sudden death, were too much for her nervous system, and my wife was soon prostrated. I felt dissatisfied with the course pursued by this physician. My confidence in his skill was shaken, and I could not employ him a second time. I called another to my suffering wife. This second physician gave her a liberal dose of opium, which he said would relieve her pains, quiet her nerves, and give her rest, which she much needed. The opium stupefied her. She slept, and nothing could arouse her from the death-like stupor. Her pulse and heart at times throbbed violently, and then grew more and more feeble in their action, until she ceased to breathe. Thus she died without giving her family one look of recognition. This second death seemed more than we could endure. We all sorrowed deeply but I was agonized and could not be comforted.

My daughter was next afflicted. Grief, anxiety and watching, had overtasked her powers of endurance, and her strength gave way, and she was brought upon a bed of suffering. I have now lost confidence in both the physicians I had employed. Another physician was recommended to me as being successful in treating the sick. And although he lived at a distance, I was determined to obtain his services.

This third physician professed to understand my daughter's case. He said that she was greatly debilitated, and that her nervous system was deranged, and that fever was upon her, which could be controlled, but that it would take time to bring her up from her present state of debility. He expressed perfect confidence in his ability to raise her. He gave her powerful medicine to break up the fever. This was accomplished. But as the fever left, the case assumed more alarming features, and grew more complicated. As the symptoms changed, the medicines were varied to meet the case. While under the influence of new medicines she would, for a time, appear revived, which would flatter our hopes, that she would get well, only to make our disappointment more bitter as she became worse.

The physician's last resort was calomel. For some time she seemed to be between life and death. She was thrown into convulsions. As these most distressing spasms ceased, we were aroused to the painful fact that her intellect was weakened. She began slowly to improve, although still a great sufferer. Her limbs were crippled as the effect of the powerful poisons which she had taken. She lingered a few years a helpless, pitiful sufferer, and died in much agony.

After this sad relation the father looked imploringly to the physician, and entreated him to save his only remaining child. The physician looked sad and anxious, but made no prescription. He arose to leave, saying that he would call the next day.

The next day: The physician was in the sick room, standing by the bedside of the afflicted daughter. Again he left the room without giving medicine. The father, when in the presence of the physician alone seemed deeply moved, and he inquired impatiently, "Do you intend to do nothing? Will you leave my only daughter to die?"

The physician said, "I have listened to the sad history of the death of your much loved wife, and your two children, and have learned from your own lips that all three have died while in the care of physicians, while taking medicines prescribed and administered by their hands. Medicine has not saved your loved ones, and as a physician I solemnly believe that none of them need, or ought to have died. They could have recovered if they had not been so drugged that nature was enfeebled by abuse, and finally crushed." He stated decidedly to the agitated father "I cannot give medicine to your daughter. I shall only seek to assist nature in her efforts, by removing every obstruction, and then leave nature to recover the exhausted energies of the system." He placed in the father's hand a few directions which he enjoined upon him to follow closely.

"Keep the patient free from excitement, and every influence calculated to depress. Her attendants should be cheerful and hopeful. She should have a simple diet, and should be allowed plenty of pure soft water to drink. Bathe frequently in pure soft water followed by gentle rubbing. Let the light, and air, be freely admitted into her room. She must have quiet, and undisturbed rest."

The father slowly read the prescription, and wondered at the few simple directions it contained, and seemed doubtful of any good resulting from such simple means. Said the physician, "You have had sufficient confidence in my skill to place the life of your daughter in my hands. Withdraw not your confidence. I will visit your daughter daily, and direct you in the management of her case. Follow my directions with confidence, and I trust in a few weeks to present her to you in a much better condition of health, if not fully restored."

The father looked sad and doubtful, but submitted to the decision of the physician. He feared that his daughter must die if she had no medicine.

A few days later: I was brought again into the sick room…the daughter was sitting by the side of her father, cheerful and happy, with the glow of health upon her countenance. The father was looking upon her with happy satisfaction, his countenance speaking the gratitude of his heart, that his only child was spared to him. Her physician entered, and after conversing with the father and child for a short time, arose to leave. He addressed the father, thus,— "I present to you your daughter restored to health. I gave her no medicine that I might leave her with an unbroken constitution. Medicine never could have accomplished this. Medicine deranges nature's fine machinery, and breaks down the constitution, and kills, but never cures. Nature alone possesses the restorative powers. She alone can build up her exhausted energies, and repair the injuries she has received by inattention to her fixed laws."

He then asked the father if he was satisfied with his manner of treatment. The happy father expressed his heartfelt gratitude, and perfect satisfaction, saying,—"I have learned a lesson I shall never forget. It was painful, yet it is of priceless value. I am now convinced that my wife and children need not have died. Their lives were sacrificed while in the hands of physicians by their poisonous drugs."

Selected Messages Book 2, pages 443-448

Story of a Young Lady Treated with (Strychnine) Nux Vomica

Another scene was then presented before me. I was brought into the presence of a female, apparently about thirty years of age. A physician was standing by her, and reporting, that her nervous system was deranged, that her blood was impure, and moved sluggishly, and that her stomach was in a cold, inactive condition. He said that he would give her active remedies which would soon improve her condition. He gave her a powder from a vial upon which was written, Nux Vomica. I watched to see what effect this would have upon the patient. It appeared to act favorably. Her condition seemed better. She was animated, and even seemed cheerful and active.

A few days later: The patient had appeared better under the influence of nux vomica. She was sitting up, folding a shawl closely around her, and complaining of chilliness. The air in the room was impure. It was heated and had lost its vitality. Almost every crevice where the pure air could enter was guarded to protect the patient from a sense of painful chilliness, which was especially felt in the back of the neck and down the spinal column. If the door was left ajar, she seemed nervous and distressed, and entreated that it should be closed, for she was cold. She could not bear the least draught of air from the door or windows. A gentleman of intelligence stood looking pityingly upon her, and said to those present,—"This is the second result of nux vomica. It is especially felt upon the nerves, and it affects the whole nervous system. There will be, for a time, increased forced action upon the nerves. But as the strength of this drug is spent, there will be chilliness, and prostration. Just to that degree that it excites and enlivens, will be the deadening, benumbing results following."

A few days later, when seen again: She was being supported by two attendants, from her chair to her bed. She had nearly lost the use of her limbs. The spinal nerves were partially paralyzed, and the limbs had lost their power to bear the weight of the person.

She coughed distressingly, and breathed with difficulty. She was laid upon the bed, and soon lost her hearing, and seeing, and thus she lingered awhile, and died. The gentleman before mentioned looked sorrowfully upon the lifeless body, and said to those present,—"Witness the mildest and protracted influence of nux vomica upon the human system.

At its introduction, the nervous energy was excited to extraordinary action to meet this drug-poison. This extra excitement was followed by prostration, and the final result has been paralysis of the nerves. This drug does not have the same effect upon all. Some who have powerful constitutions can recover from abuses to which they may subject the system.

While others, whose hold of life is not as strong, who possess enfeebled constitutions, have never recovered from receiving into the system even one dose, and many die from no other cause than the effects of one portion of this poison. Its effects are always tending to death. The condition the system is in, at the time these poisons are received into it, determine the life of the patient. Nux vomica can cripple, paralyze, destroy health forever, but it never cures."

Selected Messages Book 2, pages 445-449

Inflammation of the Bowels Healed with Charcoal

A brother was taken sick with inflammation of the bowels and bloody dysentery. The man was not a careful health reformer, but indulged his appetite. We were just preparing to leave Texas, where we had been laboring for several months, and we had carriages prepared to take away this brother and his family, and several others who were suffering from malarial fever.

My husband and I thought we would stand this expense rather than have the heads of several families die and leave their wives and children unprovided for. Two or three were taken in a large spring wagon on spring mattresses.

But this man who was suffering from inflammation of the bowels, sent for me to come to him. My husband and I decided that it would not do to move him. Fears were entertained that mortification had set in. Then the thought came to me like a communication from the Lord, to take pulverized charcoal, put water upon it, and give this water to the sick man to drink, putting bandages of the charcoal over the bowels and stomach.

We were about one mile from the city of Dennison, but the sick man's son went to a blacksmith's shop, secured the charcoal, and pulverized it, and then used it according to the directions given. The result was that in half an hour there was a change for the better. We had to go on our journey and leave the family be-hind, but what was our surprise the following day to see their wagon overtake us. The sick man was lying in a bed in the wagon. The blessing of God had worked with the simple means used

Letter 182, 1899

A Feverish Young Man Treated with Calomel

My attention was then called to still another case. I was introduced into the sick room of a young man who was in a high fever. A physician was standing by the bedside of the sufferer with a portion of medicine taken from a vial upon which was written Calomel. He administered this chemical poison, and a change seemed to take place, but not for the better.

A few days later: The third case was again presented before me. It was that of the young man to whom was administered calomel. He was a great sufferer. His lips were dark and swollen. His gums were inflamed. His tongue was thick and swollen, and the saliva was running from his mouth in large quantities. The intelligent gentleman before mentioned looked sadly upon the sufferer, and said,—"This is the influence of mercurial preparations. This young man had remaining, sufficient nervous energy, to commence a warfare upon this intruder, this drug-poison to attempt to expel it from the system. Many have not sufficient life-forces left to arouse to action, and nature is overpowered and ceases her efforts, and the victim dies."

A few days later: The third case was again presented before me, that of the young man to whom had been administered calomel. He was a pitiful sufferer. His limbs were crippled, and he was greatly deformed. He stated that his sufferings were beyond description, and life was to him a great burden. The gentleman whom I have repeatedly mentioned, looked upon the sufferer with sadness and pity, and said,—"This is the effect of calomel. It torments the system as long as there is a particle left in it. It ever lives, not losing its properties by its long stay in the living system. It inflames the joints, and often sends rottenness into the bones. It frequently manifests itself in tumors, ulcers, and cancers, years after it has been introduced into the system."

Selected Messages Book 2, pages 445-449

A Young Lady in Great Pain, Treated with Opium

I was then shown still another case. It was that of a female, who seemed to be suffering much pain. A physician stood by the bedside of the patient, and was administering medicine, taken from a vial, upon which was written, Opium. At first this drug seemed to affect the mind. She talked strangely, but finally became quiet and slept.

A few days later: She had awakened from her sleep much prostrated. Her mind was distracted. She was impatient and irritable, finding fault with her best friends, and imagining that they did not try to relieve her sufferings. She became frantic, and raved like a maniac. The gentleman before mentioned looked sadly upon the sufferer, and said to those present,—"This is the second result from taking opium."

Her physician was called. He gave her an increased dose of opium which quieted her ravings, yet made her very talkative and cheerful. She was at peace with all around

31

her, and expressed much affection for acquaintances, as well as her relatives. She soon grew drowsy and fell into a stupefied condition. The gentleman mentioned above, solemnly said,—"Her conditions of health are no better now than when she was in her frantic ravings. She is decidedly worse.

This drug-poison, opium, gives temporary relief from pain, but does not remove the cause of pain. It only stupefies the brain, rendering it incapable of receiving impressions from the nerves. While the brain is thus insensible, the hearing, the taste, and sight are affected. When the influence of opium wears off, and the brain arouses from its state of paralysis, the nerves, which had been cut off from communication with the brain, shriek out louder than ever the pains in the system, because of the additional outrage the system has sustained in receiving this poison.

Every additional drug given to the patient, whether it be opium, or some other poison, will complicate the case, and make the patient's recovery more hopeless. The drugs given to stupefy, whatever they may be, derange the nervous system. An evil, simple in the beginning, which nature aroused herself to overcome, and which she would have done had she been left to herself, has been made ten-fold worse by drug-poisons being introduced into the system, which is a destructive disease of itself, forcing into extraordinary action the remaining life-forces to war against and overcome the drug-intruder."

A few days later: The fourth case was again presented before me—the patient to whom opium had been administered. Her countenance was sallow, and her eyes were restless and glassy. Her hands shook as if palsied, and she seemed to be greatly excited, imagining that all present were leagued against her. Her mind was a complete wreck, and she raved in a pitiful manner. The physician was summoned, and seemed to be unmoved at these terrible exhibitions.

He gave the patient a more powerful portion of opium, which he said would set her all right. Her ravings did not cease until she became thoroughly intoxicated. She then passed into a deathlike stupor. The gentleman mentioned, looked upon the patient and said sadly,— "Her days are numbered. The efforts nature has made have been so many times overpowered by this poison, that the vital forces are exhausted by being repeatedly induced to unnatural action to rid the system of this poisonous drug. Nature's efforts are about to cease, and then the patient's suffering life will end."

Selected Messages Book 2, pages 445-449

Willie White Healed by the Great Physician

In the winter of 1864, my Willie was suddenly and violently brought down with lung fever. We had just buried our oldest son with this disease, and were very anxious in regard to Willie, fearing that he, too, might die. We decided that we would not send for a physician, but do the best we could with him ourselves by the use of water, and entreat the Lord in behalf of the child. We called in a few, who had faith to unite their prayers with ours. We had a sweet assurance of God's presence and blessing.

The next day Willie was very sick. He was wandering. He did not seem to see or hear me when I spoke to him. His heart had no regular beat, but was in a constant agitated flutter. We continued to look to God in his behalf, and to use water freely upon his head and a compress constantly upon his lungs and soon he seemed as rational as ever. He suffered severe pain in his right side, and could not lie upon it for a moment. This pain we subdued with cold water compresses, varying the temperature of the water according to the degree of the fever. We were very careful to keep his hands and feet warm.

We expected the crisis would come the seventh day. We had but little rest during his sickness, and were obliged to give him up into other's care the fourth and fifth nights. My husband and myself the fifth day felt very anxious. The child raised fresh blood and coughed considerably. My husband spent much time in prayer. We left our child in careful hands that night. Before retiring my husband, prayed long and earnestly. Suddenly his burden of prayer left him, and it seemed as though a voice spoke to him, and said, 'Go lie down, I will take care of the child'.

I had retired sick, and could not sleep for anxiety for several hours. I felt pressed for breath. Although sleeping in a large chamber, I arose and opened the door into a large hall, and was at once relieved, and soon slept. I dreamed that an experienced physician was standing by my child, watching every breath, with one hand over his heart, and with the other feeling his pulse. He turned to us and said, 'The crisis has passed. He has seen his worst night. He will now come up speedily for he has not the injurious influence of drugs to recover from. Nature has nobly done her work to rid the system of impurities.' I related to him my worn-out condition, my pressure for breath, and the relief obtained by opening the door.

Said he, 'That which gave you relief will also relieve your child. He needs air. You have kept him too warm. The heated air coming from a stove is injurious, and were it not for the air coming in at the crevices of the windows, would be poisonous and destroy life. Stove heat destroys the vitality of the air, and weakens the lungs. The child's lungs have been weakened by the room being kept too warm. Sick persons are debilitated by disease, and need all the invigorating air that they can bear to strengthen the vital organs to resist disease. And yet in most cases, air and light are excluded from the sick room at the very time when most needed, as though dangerous enemies.'

This dream and my husband's experience were a consolation to us both. We found in the morning that our boy had passed a restless night. He seemed to be in a high fever until noon. Then the fever left him, and he appeared quite well, except weak. He had eaten but one small cracker through his five days sickness. He came up rapidly, and has had better health than he has had for several days before. This experience is valuable to us.

Facts of Faith, pages 151-153

Additional Stories of Health Regained

Ever since we came into this missionary field we have been engaged in the work truly called Medical Missionary work. In this work we have seen the marked working of the Holy Spirit of God in the restoration of the sick. We have seen the wonderful works of God upon the hearts of men who were using tobacco and drinking liquor.

We have seen the power of God accomplishing the transformation of character, and individuals have been tested and proved and brought out of bondage into the liberty of the Gospel, and they are converted men and women. They find in Christ Jesus all that is satisfying. We see such great things accomplished that our hearts are humbled before God. The redemption and restoration of the soul is not our work but the Lord's work. It is the work of Jesus Christ, the Life-giver.

The cause we knew not we have searched out. There are whole families that this work has been instrumental in saving. This is Medical Missionary work. We had no hospital, but we used our own home as a place to which could be taken the sick and suffering, that they might be restored and saved. We have used our means to aid these people to get homes—a piece of land, and a house to live in.

In one case there was a family at Parametta, consisting of father and mother and ten children. The father was a mechanic and came to work upon the meeting house and school building and brought his three eldest boys. The wife and mother remained at home taking care of seven children until a place could be made for her. We let them occupy a small house of mine, which we furnished, so that they could keep house for themselves.

One of the boys who came with the father was a cripple, using crutches, and he cooked while the others worked. This boy is thirteen years old, and had been troubled with a knee-swelling for five years. For eleven months he was confined to his bed under the care of a physician. Sister McEnterfer had treated him with water compresses and pulverized charcoal, until the inflammation had been relieved. He was so much better that he laid aside his crutches, and attended to the cooking, as has been mentioned. But this was too much, and the knee troubled him again. It was necessary to give him a thorough course of treatment, so we took him into my own house and gave him constant care. There was a large swelling under the knee, which he called his 'egg.' This swelling was opened and discharged freely, and from it were taken pieces of bone.

What power there is in water! He improved rapidly, and he was given light work,—copying letters in the letter-book, learning to write on the type-writer and other things. We now send him to school. We board and clothe him and his father pays his tuition. We keep him for the benefit we may do the boy and he is good material to work upon. The father and mother cannot express their gratitude; for physicians, who had previously examined and treated the boy, had told them that he would be a cripple for life. The parents now look upon the boy—active and healthy, and you can judge how they feel. This is our field for missionary work.

We have helped them to get a piece of land, and the family is now united, rejoicing in a home of their own. They have a temporary house composed of a tent, the bark of trees, and corrugated iron roofing. They will soon be able to build a humble cottage of their own. The father is a carpenter, and the two eldest sons work with him.

The mother, discouraged and overworked, had given up trying to be a Christian, but her heart has broken before

God, because we have brought hope and courage to the whole family.

This boy is the third case of terribly injured limbs which have been cured by simple remedies. In each case they have been pronounced incurable by physicians. These cases have been maltreated, and it was thought that blood-poisoning had set in, in two cases. Sister McEnterfer took these cases and treated them with great pains-taking effort for weeks.

In one case we made a hospital of our home, taking care of the boy and his aunt who came with him, while the case was being treated. Sister McEnterfer accepts nothing for her labor, for I want all to know that we do this for the love of God. Case after case has received relief where physicians have failed, after charging enormous sums for their services, sometimes twenty-five and fifty dollars for a visit. In their extremity these poor souls have sent for Sister McEnterfer, and days and nights she has been five and six miles on horse-back, in the bush, where no carriage could go.

I might tell of reformations in families. The history of breaking off from tobacco and tea and coffee. I could tell of many instances where such have been truly converted, and are now standing firm for health reform. One, a fisherman and boat-maker, smoked his pipe and drank his tea even after he went to bed. He was a tea-inebriate. It took time; but he was converted. He listened to Bible readings given in certain houses and learned the truth from the Bible. The health-reform was taught and he was lead along step by step. The man carries the unmistakable marks that the Lord has wrought in his behalf. Many families have cast away tobacco and tea and coffee and liquor, and the ministry of the Word has been brought home to their hearts and convicted them of sin and righteousness and judgment.

One man, who, in prosperous times, was a well-to-do livery-man, became sick and poor, and the whole family, numbering eight, were all sick with influenza. A young man who had learned lessons in the Health Home, nursed the father, and Sister McEnterfer cared for the mother and the children, and all recovered. The father and mother came to our meetings, were convicted, and both were converted; and the father threw his pipe into the fire. When his wife saw this she cried most heartily. 'Are you feeling bad because I broke my pipe?' She said, 'Oh, no; but I thought when my family was supported by the washings I was taking from place to place, I had to give of my little to buy tobacco. Why did you not do this before' Said he, 'Wife, I was not before understanding the sinfulness of tobacco using, and liquor and tea drinking; but I will not grieve you anymore. If Brother and Sister White will give me work to do I will earn money now to support my wife and children.' He has worked steadily for one year, and he says, 'I look at myself and say: Is this Hungerford? I really scarcely know myself,—eating proper food and enjoying physical strength,—I am coming up from being sick and discouraged, and work like a strong man.'

The Gospel Herald, October 1, 1899

What Should Be Done About Drugs

Knowledge and Education Needed

Knowledge is what is needed. Drugs are too often promised to restore health, and the poor sick are so thoroughly drugged with quinine, morphine, or some strong health-and-life-destroying [medicine], that nature may never make sufficient protest, but give up the struggle; and they may continue their wrong habits with hopeful impunity.

Manuscript Releases, Volume 15

Thousands need to be educated patiently, kindly, tenderly, but decidedly, that nine-tenths of their complaints are created by their own course of action. The more they introduce drugs into the system, the more certainly do they interfere with the laws of nature and bring about the very difficulties they drug themselves to avoid.

Manuscript Releases, Volume 15

The only hope of better things is in the education of the people in right principles. Let physicians teach the people that restorative power is not in drugs, but in nature. Disease is an effort of nature to free the system from conditions that result from a violation of the laws of health. In case of sickness, the cause should be ascertained. Unhealthful conditions should be changed, wrong habits corrected. Then nature is to be assisted in her effort to expel impurities and to reestablish right conditions in the system.

Ministry of Healing, Page 127

From beginning to end, the crime of tobacco using, of opium and drug medication, has its origin in perverted knowledge. It is through plucking and eating of poisonous fruit, through the intricacies of names that the common people do not understand, that thousands and ten thousands of lives are lost. This great knowledge, supposed by men to be so wonderful, God did not mean that man should have. They are using the poisonous productions that Satan himself has planted to take the place of the tree of life, whose leaves are for the healing of the nations. Men are dealing in liquors and narcotics that are destroying the human family.

Temperance, page 75

We are health reformers. Physicians should have wisdom and experience, and be thorough health reformers. Then they will be constantly educating by precept and example their patients from drugs. For they well know that the use of drugs may produce for the time being favorable results, but will implant in the system that which will cause great difficulties hereafter, which they may never recover from during their lifetime. Nature must have a chance to do her work.

Medical Ministry, pages 224-225

Feeling existed in regard to the method that was used at the Retreat under Dr. A's directions. Dr. A, with the utmost confidence and assurance, extolled the Regular practice, and depreciated the practice of Homeopathy, and made the most extravagant statements in regard to the Regular practice. Some might take these statements as verity and

41

truth, but I knew that they were not correct; for the practice of both systems and their results had been laid open before me, and I knew that the statements that he made were not correct. But this is due to the narrow cut of the mind of the man. The system in which he has been educated he regards as the best of all methods. The Lord regards all this talk just as He regards the talk of the Pharisees,—as the invention and tradition of men.

All those who receive their education from the Regular school, and are molded by the spirit of the educators, generally act out the impressions they have received from their instructors, and denounce every other system as Satanic. Is this the way of the Lord? If the priests and Pharisees kept the way of the Lord, then Dr. A's ideas are correct. The use of drugs in our institutions, to the extent to which they are used, is a libel upon the name of hygienic institutions for the treatment of the sick. The physicians need to be converted on this point as decidedly as the sinner needs the converting power of God on life and character in order to become a pure- hearted Christian. Let the students who go to obtain a medical education at the Medical Institute of our land, learn all that they possibly can of the principles of life, but let them discard error, and not become bigots, I would not speak thus plainly, unless I felt that it was necessary.

Manuscript Releases, Volume 20

Faith—not Drugs—is the Answer

Those who see Christ by living faith, those who abide in Him, will have power to work miracles for His glory. This is why the physicians and nurses in our medical institutions should be those who abide in Christ; for though their connection with the heavenly Physician their patients will be blessed. These God-fearing workers will have no used for poisonous drugs. They will use the natural agencies that God had given for the restoration of the sick. Time and again I have told the workers in our sanitariums that from the light that God has given me, I know that they need not lose one patient suffering from a fever, if they take the case in hand in time and use rational methods of treatment instead of drugs...

When we are willing to have our own minds unsoldered, and re-soldered by the melting influences of the Spirit of God, we shall understand with new enlightenment Christ's instruction to us as recorded in the fourteenth, fifteenth, sixteenth, and seventeenth chapters of John. O how great are the possibilities that He has placed within our reach! He says, "Whatsoever ye shall ask the Father in my name, he will give it you." He promises to come to us a Comforter to bless us. Why do we not believe these promises? That which we lack in faith we make up by the use of drugs. Let us give up the drugs, believing that Jesus does not desire us to be sick, and that if we live according to the principles of health reform, He will keep us well.

Manuscript Releases, Volume 19

Drugs are the Easy Way Out

The question is, Will they preserve the principles of hygiene, or will they use the easier method of using drugs, to take the place of treating diseases without resorting to drug medication? There could be many hygienic institutions in all parts of our world, if there were plenty of means and plenty of persons who had the qualifications to manage such institutions.

Manuscript Releases, Volume 15

Drugs are not Part of God's Plan

The use of drugs is not in accordance with God's plan. Physicians should understand how to treat the sick through the use of nature's remedies. Pure air, pure water, healthful exercise should be employed in the treatment of the sick...

Many indulge in unhealthful practices until the physical vitality is undermined, and the mental and moral powers are enfeebled. When they fall a prey to disease they resort to drugs, and if these afford them temporary relief, they seem to be satisfied to continue in transgression. They do not bring their habits and practices in review to see what is wrong, and correct the evils by removing the cause. As the drugs are a mere stimulant, after a time they realize that they are in a worse condition than before they used the remedies. To use drugs while continuing evil habits, is certainly inconsistent, and greatly dishonors God by dishonoring the body which He has made. Yet for all this, stimulants and drugs continue to be prescribed, and freely used by human beings, while the hurtful indulgences that produced the disease are not discarded. They use tea, coffee, tobacco, opium, wine, beer, and other stimulants, and give to nature a false support.

Manuscript Releases, Volume 16

We Should Avoid All Poisons

God's servants should not administer medicines which they know will leave behind injurious effects upon the system, even if they do relieve present suffering. Every poisonous preparation in the vegetable and mineral kingdoms, taken into the system, will leave its wretched influence, affecting the liver and lungs, and deranging the system generally.

Spiritual Gifts Vol. IV., page 140

Nothing should be put into the human system that will leave a baleful influence behind.

Medical Ministry, page 228

The simplest remedies may assist nature, and leave no baleful effects after their use.

Letter 82, 1897 (To Dr. J.H. Kellogg)

Reducing the Use of Drugs

In their practice, the physicians should seek more and more to lessen the use of drugs instead of increasing it...Thus our people, who had been taught to avoid drugs in almost every form, were receiving a different education.

Letter 26a, 1889

Trust not to your own human wisdom. Trust not in poisonous drugs, that will interfere with nature's work, and leave their cruel trail behind. Work away from drugs, and never, never advise one under your influence to go to Ann Arbor or any place to obtain the education supposed to be essential for the perfection of the medical practitioner. The stamp left upon them by such places is almost ineffaceable. Educate, educate, educate, by placing yourself and others in the closest connection with the greatest Healer the world has ever known.

Manuscript Releases, Volume Twenty-One

Our institutions are established that the sick may be treated by hygienic methods, discarding almost entirely the use of drugs.

Temperance, page 88

The first labors of a physician should be to educate the sick and suffering in the very course they should pursue to prevent disease. The greatest good can be done by our trying to enlighten the minds of all we can obtain access to, as to the best course for them to pursue to prevent sickness and suffering, and broken constitutions, and premature death. But those who do not care to undertake work that taxes their physical and mental powers will be ready to prescribe drug medication, which lays a foundation in the human organism for a twofold greater evil than that which they claim to have relieved.

A physician who has the moral courage to imperil his reputation in enlightening the understanding by plain facts, in showing the nature of disease and how to prevent it, and the dangerous practice of resorting to drugs, will have an uphill business, but he will live and let live. He will not use his powerful drug medication, because of the knowledge he has acquired by studying books. He will, if a reformer, talk plainly in regard to the false appetites and ruinous self-indulgence, in dressing, in eating and drinking, in overtaxing to do a large amount of work in a given time, which has a ruinous influence upon the temper, the physical and mental powers...

Right and correct habits, intelligently and perseveringly practiced, will be removing the cause for disease, and the strong drugs need not be resorted to. Many go on from step to step with their unnatural indulgences, which is bringing in just as unnatural {a} condition of things as possible.

Medical Ministry, pages 221- 222

Drug medication, as it is generally practiced, is a curse. Educate away from drugs. Use them less and less, and depend more upon hygienic agencies; then nature will respond to God's physicians—pure air, pure water, proper exercise, a clear conscience. Those who persist in the use of tea, coffee, and flesh meats will feel the need of drugs, but many might recover without one grain of medicine if they would obey the laws of health. Drugs need seldom be used.

Counsels on Health, page 261

Do not administer drugs. True, drugs may not be as dangerous wisely administered as they usually are, but in the hands of many will be hurtful to the Lord's property.

Letter 3, 1884

Educate people in the laws of life so that they may know how to preserve health. The efforts actually put forth at present are not meeting the mind of God. Drug medication is a curse to this enlightened age.

Educate away from drugs. Use them less and less, and depend more upon hygienic agencies; then nature will respond to God's physicians,— pure air, pure water, proper exercise, a clear conscience.

Many might recover without one grain of medicine, if they would live out the laws of health. Drugs need seldom be used. It will require earnest, patient, protracted effort to establish the work and to carry it forward upon hygienic principles. But let fervent prayer and faith be combined with your efforts, and you will succeed. By this work you will be teaching the patients, and others also, how to take care of themselves when sick, without resorting to the use of drugs.

Medical Ministry, pages 259-260

The use of drugs in our institutions, to the extent to which they are used, is a libel upon the name of hygienic institutions for the treatment of the sick.

Manuscript Releases Volume Twenty, page 394

We wish to build a sanitarium {in Australia} where maladies may be cured by nature's own provisions, and where the people may be taught how to treat themselves when sick; where they will learn to eat temperately of wholesome food, and be educated to refuse all narcotics,— tea, coffee, fermented wines, and stimulants of all kinds, — and to discard the flesh of dead animals.

Selected Messages Book 2, page 281

Our sanitariums are one of the most successful means of reaching all classes of people. Christ is no longer in this world in person, to go through our cities and towns and villages healing the sick. He has commissioned us to carry forward the medical missionary work that He began; and in this work we are to do our very best. Institutions for the care of the sick are to be established, where men and women may be placed under the care of God-fearing medical missionaries and be treated without drugs. To these institutions will come those who have brought disease on themselves by improper habits of eating and drinking. These are to be taught the principles of healthful living. They are to be taught the value of self- denial and self-restraint. They are to be provided with a simple, wholesome, palatable diet and are to be cared for by wise physicians and nurses.

Our sanitariums are the right hand of the gospel, opening doors whereby suffering humanity may be reached with the glad tidings of healing through Christ. In these institutions the sick may be taught to commit their cases to the Great Physician, who will co-operate with their earnest efforts to regain health, bringing to them healing of soul as well as healing of body.

Counsels on Health, page 212

The light given me was that a sanitarium should be established, and that in it drug medication should be discarded, and simple, rational methods of treatment employed for the healing of disease. In this institution people were to be taught how to dress, breathe, and eat properly—how to prevent sickness by proper habits of living.

Counsels on Diet and Foods, page 303

It would have been better if, from the first, all drugs had been kept out of our sanitariums, and use had been made of such simple remedies as are found in pure water, pure air, sunlight, and some of the simple herbs growing in the field. These would be just as efficacious as the drugs used under mysterious names, and concocted by human science, and they would leave no injurious effects in the system.

Lead them [the people] away from drug medication, educating them and training them that drugs kill more than they cure. This matter is presented to me so frequently, that I cannot hold my peace upon this subject. The use of poisonous drugs is coming more and more into practice among our people. The light which the Lord has given me is, that institutions should be established to do away with drugs, and use God's agencies; that instruction should be given daily upon this subject. But God's ways and instruction have not been heeded, therefore not one twentieth part of the good has been accomplished which might have been if Christian physicians had heeded the admonitions and the counsel of the Most High.

Manuscript Releases, Volume 20

As matters have been opened to me from time to time, as I have been conducted through the rooms of the sick in the Sanitarium and out of the Sanitarium, I have seen that the physicians of the Sanitarium, by practicing drug medication, have lost many cases that need not have died if they had left their drugs out of the sick room. Cases have been lost that, had the physicians left off entirely their drug treatment, had they put their wits to work, and wisely and persistently used the Lord's own remedies, plenty of air and water,—the fever cases that have been lost would have recovered. The reckless use of those things that should be discarded has decided the case of the sick.

I will not educate or sustain the use of drugs...After seeing so much harm done by the administering of drugs, I cannot use them, and cannot testify in their favor. I must be true to the light given me by the Lord.

The treatment we gave when the Sanitarium was first established required earnest labor to combat disease. We did not use drug concoctions; we followed hygienic methods. This work was blessed by God. It was a work in which the human instrumentality could cooperate with God in saving life. There should be nothing put into the human system that would leave its baleful influence behind. And to carry out the light on this subject, to practice hygienic treatment, and to educate on altogether different lines of treating the sick, was the reason given me why we should have sanitariums established in various localities. I have been pained when many students have been encouraged to go Ann Arbor, to receive an education in the use of drugs. The light which I have received has placed an altogether different complexion on the use made of drugs than is given at Ann Arbor or at the Sanitarium. We must become enlightened on these subjects.

Manuscript Releases, Volume 21

The light was given that we should have a sanitarium, a health institution, which was to be established right among us. This was the means God was to use in bringing His people to a right understanding in regard to health reform.

It was also to be the means by which we were to gain access to those not of our faith. We were to have an institution where the sick could be relieved of suffering, and that without drug medication. God declared that He Himself would go before His people in this work.

Counsels on Health, page 531

When you understand physiology in its truest sense, your drug bills will be very much smaller, and finally you will cease to deal out drugs at all. The physician who depends upon drug medication in his practice, shows that he does not understand the delicate machinery of the human organism. He is introducing into the system a seed crop that will never lose its destroying properties through the lifetime. I tell you this because I dare not withhold it. Christ paid too much for man's redemption to have his body so ruthlessly treated as it has been by drug medication.

Years ago the Lord revealed to me that institutions should be established for treating the sick without drugs. Man is God's property, and the ruin that has been made of the living habitation, the suffering caused by the seeds of death sown in the human system, are an offense to God.

Medical Ministry, page 229

You should avoid the use of drugs and carefully observe the laws of health. If you regard your life you should eat plain food, prepared in the simplest manner, and take more physical exercise. Each member of the family needs the benefits of health reform. But drugging should be forever abandoned; for while it does not cure any malady, it enfeebles the system, making it more susceptible to disease.

Testimonies, Vol. 5, page 311

Our sanitariums are established as institutions where patients and helpers may serve God. We desire to encourage as many as possible to act their part individually in living healthfully. We desire to encourage the sick to discard the use of drugs, and to substitute the simple remedies provided by God, as they are found in water, in pure air, in exercise, and in general hygiene.

Manuscript Releases, Volume One

In their practice, the physicians should seek more and more to lessen the use of drugs instead of increasing it. When Dr. A came to the Health Retreat, she laid aside her knowledge and practice of hygiene, and administered the little homeopathic doses for almost every ailment. This was against the light God had given. Thus our people, who had been taught to avoid drugs in almost every form, were receiving a different education. I was obliged to tell her that this practice of depending upon medicine, whether in large or small doses, was not in accordance with the principles of health reform. The Lord had in His providence given light in regard to the establishment of sanitariums where the sick should be treated upon hygienic principles. The people must be taught to depend on the Lord's remedies, pure air, pure water, simple, healthful foods...

Selected Message Book 2, page 282

Physicians have a work to do to bring about reform by educating the people, that they may understand the laws which govern their physical life. They should know how to eat properly, to work intelligently, and to dress healthfully, and should be taught to bring all their habits into harmony with the laws of life and health, and to discard drugs. There is a great work to be done. If the principles of health reform are carried out, the work will indeed be as closely allied to that of the third angel's message as the hand is to the body...

If they move in God's way, physicians of the same faith will be linked together in a strong brotherhood, aiding one another to reach the highest standard, and devise means to enlighten the people, not encouraging in the use of drugs, but leading away from drug medication. Teach the people how to prevent disease. Tell them to cease rebelling against nature's laws, and by removing every obstruction, give her a chance to put forth her very best efforts to set things right. Nature must have a fair chance to employ her healing agencies. We must make earnest efforts to reach a higher platform in regard to the methods of treating the sick. If the light which God has given prevails, if truth overcomes error, advanced steps will be taken in health reform. This must be.

Manuscript Releases, Volume 13

The Health Retreat [St. Helena Sanitarium] was established at a great cost to treat the sick without drugs. It should be conducted on hygienic principles. Drug medication should be worked away from as fast as possible, until entirely discarded. Education should be given on proper diet, dress, and exercise. Not only should our own people be educated, but those who have not received the light upon health reform should be taught how to live healthfully, according to God's order.

Counsels on Diets and Foods, page 406

I sick, I would just as soon call in a lawyer as a physician from among general practitioners. I would not touch their nostrums, to which they give Latin names. I am determined to know, in straight English, the name of everything that I introduced into my system.

Selected Messages Book 2, page 290

Last night I spent many wakeful hours in prayer. I am resolved to cast myself, body, soul, and spirit, upon the Lord. I cannot take drugs. They do me no good, but harm. I long for the blessing of the Lord. My heart goes out after God. I tremble at His word. I am encouraged as I look to Jesus and recount His loving-kindnesses: "In my distress I called upon the Lord, and cried unto my God: He heard my voice out of His temple, and my cry came before Him, even into His ears." "He brought me forth also into a large place; He delivered me, because He delighted in me." "I love the Lord, because He hath heard my voice and my supplications." This has been my experience day and night during my sickness.

Manuscript Releases Vol. 19, page 297

Drugs Should Be Discarded

Drug medication is to be discarded. On this point the conscience of the physician must ever be kept tender, and true, and clean. The inclination to use poisonous drugs, which kill, if they do not cure, needs to be guarded against.

55

Matters have been laid open before me in reference to the use of drugs. Many have been treated with drugs, and the result has been death. Our physicians, by practicing drug medication, have lost many cases that need not have died if they had left their drugs out of the sick-room.

Fever cases have been lost, when had the physicians left off entirely their drug treatment, had they put their wits to work, and wisely and persistently used the Lord's own remedies, plenty of air and water, the patients would have recovered. The reckless use of these things that should be discarded has decided the case of the sick.

Experimenting in drugs is a very expensive business. Paralysis of the brain and tongue is often the result, and the victims die an unnatural death, when, if they had been treated perseveringly with unwearied, unrelaxed diligence, with hot and cold water, hot compresses, packs and dripping sheets, they would be alive today.

Nothing should be put into the human system that will leave a baleful influence behind. And to carry out the light on this subject, to practice hygienic treatment, is the reason which has been given me for establishing sanitariums in various localities....

I have been pained when many students have been encouraged to go where they would receive an education in the use of drugs. The light I have received on the subject of drugs is altogether different from the use made of them at these schools or at the sanitariums. We must become enlightened on these subjects.

The intricate names given medicines are used to cover up the matter, so that none will know what is given them as remedies unless they consult a dictionary....

Patients are to be supplied with good, wholesome food; total abstinence from all intoxicating drinks is to be observed; drugs are to be discarded, and rational methods of treatment followed. The patients must not be given alcohol, tea, coffee, or drugs; for these always leave traces of evil behind them. By observing these rules, many who have been given up by the physicians may be restored to health.

In this work the human and divine instrumentalities can cooperate in saving life, and God will add His blessing. Many suffering ones not of our faith will come to our institutions to receive treatment. Those whose health has been ruined by sinful indulgence, and who have been treated by physicians till the drugs administered have no effect, will come; and they will be benefited.

The Lord will bless institutions conducted in accordance with His plans. He will cooperate with every physician who faithfully and conscientiously engages in this work. He will enter the rooms of the sick. He will give wisdom to the nurses.

Medical Ministry, pages 227-229

The use of drugs has resulted in far more harm than good; and should our physicians who claim to believe the truth almost entirely dispense with medicine, and faithfully practice alone the lines of the principles of hygiene, using nature's remedies, far greater success would attend their efforts. The duties and qualifications of a physician are not small.

Special Testimonies
Book D, pages 270- 271

Simple Remedies are Best

The Call to Use Simple Remedies

Thousands who are afflicted might recover their health, if, instead of depending upon the drugstore for their life, they would discard all drugs, and live simply, without using tea, coffee, liquor, or spices, which irritate the stomach and leave it weak, unable to digest even simple food without stimulation. God is willing to let His light shine forth in clear, distinct rays to all who are weak and feeble.

Medical Ministry, page 229

Pure air, sunlight, abstemiousness, rest, exercise, proper diet, the use of water, trust in divine power—these are the true remedies. Every person should have a knowledge of nature's remedial agencies and how to apply them. It is essential both to understand the principles involved in the treatment of the sick and to have a practical training that will enable one rightly to use this knowledge.

Ministry of Healing, page 127

Now in regard to that which we can do for ourselves: There is a point that requires careful, thoughtful consideration. I must become acquainted with myself. I must be a learner always as to how to take care of this building, the body God has given me, that I may preserve it in the very best condition of health. I must eat those things which will be for my very best good physically, and I must take special care to have my clothing such as will conduce to a healthful circulation of the blood. 1 must not deprive myself of exercise and air. 1 must get all the sunlight that it is possible for me to obtain.

I must have wisdom to be a faithful guardian of my body. I should do a very unwise thing to enter a cool room when in a perspiration; I should show myself an unwise steward to allow myself to sit in a draught and thus expose myself so as to take cold. I should be unwise to sit with cold feet and limbs and thus drive back the blood from the extremities to the brain or internal organs. 1 should always protect my feet in damp weather.

I should eat regularly of the most healthful food which will make the best quality of blood, and I should not work intemperately if it is in my power to avoid doing so.

And when I violate the laws God has established in my being, I am to repent and reform, and place myself in the most favorable condition under the doctors God has provided, Pure air, pure water, and the healing, precious sunlight. Water can be used in many ways to relieve suffering. Draughts of clear, hot water taken before eating (half a quart more or less), will never do any harm, but will rather be productive of good.

The Place of Herbs in Rational Therapy, page 6

Your letter to me, under date Feb. 12, is received. Your question is, "Is it advisable to employ a good, Christian physician, who treats his patients on hygienic principles? In urgent cases, should we call in a worldly physician, because the sanitarium doctors are all so busy that they have no time to devote to outside practice? Some say that when the sanitarium doctors do use drugs, they give larger doses than ordinary doctors."

If the physicians are so busy that they cannot treat the sick outside of the institution, would it not be wiser for all to educate themselves in the use of simple remedies, than to venture to use drugs, that are given a long name to hide their real qualities. Why need anyone be ignorant of God's remedies,—hot water fomentations and cold and hot compresses. It is important to become familiar with the benefit of dieting in case of sickness. All should understand what to do themselves. They may call upon someone who understands nursing, but everyone should have an intelligent knowledge of the house he lives in. All should understand what to do in case of sickness...

The Paulson Collection of Ellen G. White Letters, page 14

Those who make a practice of taking drugs sin against their intelligence and endanger their whole after life. There are herbs that are harmless, the use of which will tide over many apparently serious difficulties. But if all would seek to become intelligent in regard to their bodily necessities, sickness would be rare instead of common. An ounce of prevention is worth a pound of cure.

Selected Message Book 2, page 290

I have been unable to sleep after half-past eleven at night. Many things, in figures and symbols, are passing before me. There are sanitariums in running order near Los Angeles. At one place there is an occupied building, and there are fruit trees on the sanitarium grounds. In this institution, outside the city, there is much activity.

As in the vision of the night I saw the grounds, I said, "O ye of little faith! You have lost time." There were sick in wheelchairs. There were some patients to whom the physicians had given a prescription to spend all their time outdoors during pleasant weather, in order to regain health...

While speaking, I said: "We must have sanitariums in favored places in different localities. This is God's plan. He has ordained the medical missionary work as a means of saving souls, and that which we see about us is a symbol of the work before us. We are to awaken our churches to engage interestedly in God's work, and to carry forward this branch,—the medical missionary work."

Physicians were interested in these words, and one said, as he extended his arms and waved them back and forth, "Is not this better than drugs? Aches and pains have left you without the use of medicine."

On the grounds that I saw in this vision of the night, there were shade trees, the boughs of which were hung in such a way that they formed leafy canopies somewhat the shape of tents. The sick were delighted. While some were working for diversion, others were singing. There was no dissatisfaction.

Manuscript Releases, Volume One

There are many simple herbs which, if our nurses would learn the value of, they could use in the place of drugs, and find very effective.

Letter 90, 1908

By His own working agencies He has created material which will restore the sick to health. If men would use aright the wisdom God has given them, this world would be a place resembling heaven.

Manuscript 63, 1899

We should make decided efforts to heed .the directions the Lord has given in regard to the care of the sick. They should be given every advantage possible. All the restorative agencies that the Lord has provided should he made use of in our sanitarium work.

Manuscript 19, 1911

There are many ways of practicing the healing art, but there is only one way that Heaven approves. God's remedies are the simple agencies of nature that will not tax or debilitate the system through their powerful properties. Pure air and water, cleanliness, a proper diet, purity of life, and a firm trust in God are remedies for the want of which thousands are dying; yet these remedies are going out of date because their skillful use requires work that the people do not appreciate. Fresh air, exercise, pure water, and clean, sweet premises are within the reach of all with but little expense, but drugs are expensive, both in the outlay of means and in the effect produced upon the system.

Testimonies for the Church, Volume Five, page 443

The work of the Christian physician does not end with healing the maladies of the body; his efforts should extend to the diseases of the mind, to the saving of the soul. It may not be his duty, unless asked, to present any theoretical points of truth; but he may point his patients to Christ. The lessons of the divine Teacher are ever appropriate. He should call the attention of the repining to the ever fresh tokens of the love and care of God, to His wisdom and goodness as manifested in His created works. The mind can then be led through nature up to nature's God and centered on the heaven which He has prepared for those that love Him.

The physician should know how to pray. In many cases he must increase suffering in order to save life; and whether the patient is a Christian or not, he feels greater security if he knows that his physician fears God. Prayer will give the sick an abiding confidence; and many times if their cases are borne to the Great Physician in humble trust, it will do more for them than all the drugs that can be administered.

Testimonies Vol. 5, page 443

Nature will want some assistance to bring things to their proper condition, which may be found in the simplest remedies, especially in the use of nature's own furnished remedies,—pure air, and with a precious knowledge of how to breathe; pure water, with a knowledge of how to apply it; plenty of sunlight in every room in the house if possible, and with an intelligent knowledge of what advantages are to be gained by its use. All these are powerful in their efficiency, and the patient who has obtained a knowledge of how to eat and dress healthfully, may live for comfort, for peace, for health; and will not be prevailed upon to put to his lips drugs, which, in the place of helping nature, paralyzes her powers. If the sick and suffering will do only as well as they know in regard to living out the principles of health reform perseveringly, then they will in nine cases out of ten recover from their ailments.

The feeble and suffering ones must be educated line upon line, precept upon precept, here a little and there a little, until they will have respect for and live in obedience to the law that God has made to control the human organism. Those who sin against knowledge and light, and resort to the skill of a physician in administering drugs, will be constantly losing their hold on life. The less there is of drug dosing, the more favorable will be their recovery to health. Drugs, in the place of helping nature, are constantly paralyzing her efforts.

Medical Ministry, pages 223-224

Small sanitariums are to be connected with our schools. The students are to be taught how to use nature's simple remedies in the treatment of disease. And as they learn to care for the sick, they are to be taught to act under the direction of the Lord Jesus Christ.

Review and Herald,
Sept. 9, 1902

The question of health reform is not agitated as it must and will be. A simple diet, and the entire absence of drugs, leaving nature free to recuperate the wasted energies of the body, would make our sanitariums far more effectual in restoring the sick to health.

Temperance, page 89

Institutions for the care of the sick are to be established, where men and women suffering from disease may be placed under the care of God-fearing physicians and nurses, and be treated without drugs.

Testimonies for the Church, Vol. 9, page 168

One patient, successfully treated, will have a testimony to bear of the virtue of the simple methods of treatment, the simple, healthful remedies that nature has provided, without the use of any drugs.

The Paulson Collection of Ellen G. White Letters, page 40

Drugs Not a Replacement for Temperance or Natural Remedies

In the Saviour's manner of healing, there were lessons for His disciples. On one occasion He anointed the eyes of a blind man with clay, and bade him, "Go, wash in the pool of Siloam...He went his way therefore, and washed, and came seeing." John 9:7. The cure could be wrought only by the power of the great Healer, yet Christ made use of the simple agencies of nature. While He did not give countenance to drug medication, He sanctioned the use of simple and natural remedies...

And we should teach others how to preserve and to recover health. For the sick we should use the remedies which God has provided in nature, and we should point them to Him who alone can restore. It is our work to present the sick and suffering to Christ in the arms of our faith. We should teach them to believe in the great Healer. We should lay hold on His promise, and pray for the manifestation of His power. The very essence of the gospel is restoration, and the Saviour would have us bid the sick, the hopeless, and the afflicted take hold upon His strength.

Counsels on Health, pages 30-31

Our people should become intelligent in the treatment of sickness without the aid of poisonous drugs. Many should seek to obtain the education that will enable them to combat disease in its varied forms by the most simple methods. Thousands have gone down to the grave because of the use of poisonous drugs, who might have been restored to health by simple methods of treatment. Water treatments, wisely and skillfully given, may be the means of saving many lives.

Medical Ministry page 227

In regard to the matter of prayer for the sick, many confusing ideas are advanced. One says, He who has been prayed for must walk out in faith, giving God the glory, and making use of no remedies. If he is at a health institute, he should leave it at once. I know that these ideas are wrong, and that if accepted, they would lead to many evils. On the other hand, I do not wish to say anything that might be interpreted to mean a lack of belief in the efficacy of prayer.

The path of faith lies close beside the path of presumption. It is no denial of faith to use rational remedies judiciously. Water, air, and sunshine, these are God's healing agencies. It is no denial of faith to use rational remedies judiciously. Water, air, and sunshine, these are God's healing agencies. The use of certain herbs that the

Lord has made to grow for the good of man is in harmony with the exercise of faith.

Manuscript 31, 1911

Physicians are placed in positions of temptation and danger. But they may stand firm to their allegiance if they will take hold of the strength that God offers them. He says, "Let him take hold of my strength, that he may make peace with me, and he shall make peace with me." The Lord will be the helper of every physician who will work together with Him in the effort to restore suffering humanity to health, not with drugs, but with nature's remedies. Christ is the great Physician, the wonderful Healer. He gives success to those who work in partnership with Him.

Letter 142, 1902
Bro. W.H. Jones

Nature's simple remedies will aid in recovery without leaving the deadly aftereffects so often felt by those who use poisonous drugs. They destroy the power of the patient to help himself. This power the patients are to be taught to exercise by learning to eat simple, healthful foods, by refusing to overload the stomach with a variety of foods at one meal. All these things should come into the education of the sick. Talks should be given showing how to preserve health, how to shun sickness, how to rest when rest is needed.

Selected Messages Book 2, page 281

Many parents substitute drugs for judicious nursing.

Health Reformer
Sept. 1866

Men and women use drugs of every description to counteract the results of their own misdoings. Then they charge their suffering to the providence of God, and finish the business by calling in a physician, who drugs to death the remaining forces of nature.

Manuscript 155, 1899

The use of natural remedies requires an amount of care and effort that many are not willing to give. Nature's process of healing and upbuilding is gradual, and to the impatient it seems slow. The surrender of hurtful indulgences requires sacrifice. But in the end it will be found that nature, untrammeled, does her work wisely and well. Those who persevere in obedience to her laws will reap the reward in health of body and health of mind.

Ministry of Healing, page 126-127

The Lord will heal those who believe, but He has given natural blessings for the benefit of the afflicted, and He would have these used. God could have healed Hezekiah with a word. But He heard Hezekiah's prayer, and gave directions that a bunch of figs be placed upon the diseased parts. This was done, and Hezekiah recovered. But his recovery was not instantaneous. He had not the same faith that the afflicted woman had. We need to exercise faith. To practice the use of drug medication does not harmonize with faith. Appealing to worldly physicians is dishonoring to God. Those who come to God in faith must cooperate with Him in accepting and using His heaven-sent remedies,—water, sunlight, and plenty of air.

It is of no use to have seasons of prayer for the sick, while they refuse to use the simple remedies which God has provided, and which are close by them. If there is an unsanitary condition of things in the house and about the premises, the very first thing is to take up the work that has been neglected, and cleanse and purify the house and premises, making everything sweet, that the atmosphere may not be tainted by the least offensive smell.

The Paulson Collection of Ellen G. White Letters, page 40

The drug science has been exalted, but if every bottle that comes from every such institution were done away with, there would be fewer invalids in the world today. Drug medication should never have been introduced into our institutions. There was no need of this being so, and for this very reason the Lord would have us establish an institution where He can come in and where His grace and power can be revealed. "I am the Resurrection and the Life," He declares.

The true method for healing the sick is to tell them of the herbs that grow for the benefit of man. Scientists have attached large names to these simplest preparations, but true education will lead us to teach the sick that they need not call in a doctor any more than they would call in a lawyer. They can themselves administer the simple herbs if necessary. To educate the human family that the doctor alone knows all the ills of infants and persons of every age is false teaching, and the sooner we as a people stand on the principles of health reform, the greater will be the blessing that will come to those who would do true medical work. There is a work to be done in treating the sick with water, and teaching them to make the most of the sunshine and physical exercise. Thus in simple language we may teach the people how to preserve health, how to avoid sickness. This is the work our sanitariums are called upon to do. This is true science.

Manuscript 105, 1898

A Better Diet Would Remove Much of the Need for Drugs

A simple diet, and the entire absence of drugs, leaving nature to recuperate the wasted energies of the body, would make our sanitariums more effectual in restoring the sick to health....There is need that temperance in eating, drinking, and building be practiced. There is need to educate the people in right habits of living. Put no confidence in drug medicine. If every particle of it were buried in the great ocean, I would say, Amen; for physicians are not working on a right plan. A reform is needed which will go deeper, and be more thorough.

Letter 73a, 1896
A doctor and his wife

Ill health in a variety of forms, if effect could be traced to the cause, would reveal the sure-result of flesh eating. The disuse of meats, with healthful dishes nicely prepared to take the place of flesh meats, would place a large number of the sick and suffering ones in a fair way of recovering their health, without the use of drugs. But if the physician encourages a meat-eating diet to his invalid patients, then he will make a necessity for the use of drugs...

Drugs always have a tendency to break down and destroy vital forces, and nature becomes so crippled in her efforts, that the invalid dies, not because he needed to die, but because nature was outraged. If she had been left alone, she should have put forth her highest efforts to save life and health. Nature wants none of such help as so many claim that they have given her. Lift off the burdens placed upon her, after the customs of the fashion of this age, and you will see in many cases nature will right herself. The use of drugs is not favorable or natural to the laws of life and health. The drug medication gives nature two burdens to bear, in the place of one.

Medical Ministry, pages 222-223

The diet affects both physical and moral health.

Christian Temperance and Bible Hygiene, page 79

The many dishes usually prepared for dessert should be dispensed with.

Healthful Living, page 76

There is religion in good cooking, and I question the religion of that class who are too ignorant and too careless to learn to cook.

Testimonies for the Church, Vol. 2 page 537

It is the positive duty of physicians to educate, educate, educate, by pen and voice, all who have the responsibility of preparing food for the table.

Healthful Living, page 77

Is my diet such as will bring me in a position where I can accomplish the greatest amount of good?

The Review and Herald, June 17, 1880

The Lord intends to bring his people back to live upon simple fruits, vegetables, and grains.... God provided fruit in its natural state for our first parents.

Healthful Living, page 78

Cheese should never be introduced into the stomach.

Testimonies for the Church, Vol. 2 page 68

Jesus, speaking of the cloudy pillar, gave special direction to the children of Israel, saying: "It shall be a perpetual statute for your generations throughout all your dwellings, that ye eat neither fat nor blood." "And the Lord spake unto Moses, saying, Speak unto the children of Israel, saying, Ye shall eat no manner of fat, of ox, of sheep, or of goat." "For whosoever eateth the fat of the beasts, of which men offer an offering made by fire unto the Lord, even the soul that eateth it shall be cut off from

Healthful Living, page 78

Meat is not essential for health or strength, else the Lord made a mistake when he provided food for Adam and Eve before their fall. All the elements of nutrition are contained in the fruits, vegetables, and grains.

The Review and Herald, May 8, 1883

The Lord intends to bring his people back to live upon simple fruits, vegetables, and grains. He led the children of Israel into the wilderness where they could not get a flesh diet; and he gave them the bread of heaven. "Man did eat angels' food." But they craved the flesh-pots of Egypt, and mourned and cried for flesh, notwithstanding the promise of the Lord that if they would submit to his will, he would carry them into the land of Canaan, and establish them there, a pure, holy, happy people, and that there should not be a feeble one in all their tribes; for he would take away all sickness from among them.... The Lord would have given them flesh had it been essential for their health, but he who had created and redeemed them led them through that long journey in the wilderness to educate, discipline, and train them in correct habits. The Lord understood what influence flesh eating has upon the human system. He would have a people that would, in their physical appearance, bear the divine credentials, notwithstanding their long journey.

Healthful Living, page 96

Let no meat be found at our restaurants or dining tents, but let its place be supplied with fruits, grains, and vegetables. We must practise what we preach. When sitting at a table where meat is provided, we should not make a raid on those who use it, but should let it alone ourselves; and when asked the reason for doing this, we should kindly explain why we do not use it.

The diet of animals is vegetables and grains. Must the vegetables be animalized, must they be incorporated into the system of an animal, before we get them? Must we obtain our vegetable diet by eating the flesh of dead creatures? God provided food in its natural state for our first parents. He gave Adam charge of the garden, to dress it and to care for it, saying, "To you it shall be for meat." One animal was not to destroy another animal for food.

Those who have lived upon a meat diet all their lives do not see the evil of continuing the practise, and they must be treated tenderly.

Healthful Living, page 97

One of the great errors that many insist upon is that muscular strength is dependent upon animal food. But the simple grains, fruits of the trees, and vegetables have all the nutritive properties necessary to make good blood. This a flesh diet cannot do.

Healthful Living, page 98

Speaking in support of this diet, they said that without it they were weak in physical strength. But the words of our Teacher to us were, "As a man thinketh, so is he." The flesh of dead animals was not the original food for man. Man was permitted to eat it after the flood, because all vegetation had been destroyed.... Since the flood the human race has been shortening the period of its existence. Physical, mental, and moral degeneracy is rapidly increasing in these last days.

Healthful Living, page 98

The weakness experienced on leaving off meat is one of the strongest arguments that I could present as a reason why you should discontinue its use. Those who eat meat feel stimulated after eating this food, and they suppose that they are made stronger. After they discontinue the use of meat, they may for a time feel weak, but when the system is cleansed from the effect of this diet, they no longer feel the weakness, and will cease to wish for that for which they have pleaded as essential to strength.

Healthful Living, page 98

The use of the flesh of animals tends to cause a grossness of the body.

Testimonies for the Church, page 263

When we feed on flesh, the juices of what we eat pass into the circulation. A feverish condition is created, because the animals are diseased, and by partaking of their flesh we plant the seeds of disease in our own tissue and blood. Then, when exposed to the changes of a malarious atmosphere, to prevailing epidemics and contagious diseases, these are more sensibly felt, for the system is not in a condition to resist disease.

Healthful Living, page 100

Because those who partake of animal food do not immediately feel its effects, is no evidence that it does not injure them. It may be doing its work surely upon the system, and yet the persons for the time being realize nothing of it.

How to Live, page 100

The liability to take disease is increased tenfold by meat eating.

Healthful Living, page 100

Cancers, tumors, and various other inflammatory diseases are largely caused by meat eating. From the light which God has given me, the prevalence of cancers and tumors is largely due to gross living on dead flesh.

Healthful Living, page 100

Cancers, tumors, diseases of the lungs, the liver, and the kidneys, all exist in the animals that are used for food.

Healthful Living, page 101

It is impossible for those who make free use of flesh meats to have an unclouded brain and an active intellect.

Testimonies for the Church, Vol. 2, page 62

Such a diet contaminates the blood and stimulates the lower passions. It prevents vigor of thought and enfeebles the perceptions, so that God and the truth are not understood.

Healthful Living, page 102

Disease of every type is afflicting the human family, and it is largely the result of subsisting on the diseased flesh of dead animals.

Healthful Living, page 102

There are but few animals that are free from disease. Many have been made to suffer greatly for the want of light, pure air, and wholesome food. When they are fattened, they are often confined in close stables, and are not permitted to exercise, and to enjoy free circulation of air. Many poor animals are left to breathe the poison of filth which is left in barns and stables. Their lungs will not long remain healthy while inhaling such impurities. Disease is conveyed to the liver, and the entire system of the animal is diseased. They are killed, and prepared for the market, and people eat freely of this poisonous animal food. Much disease is caused in this manner. But the people cannot be made to believe that it is the meat they have eaten which has poisoned their blood, and caused their sufferings. Many die of disease caused wholly by meat eating, yet the world does not seem to be the wiser.... It may be doing its work surely upon the system, and yet the person for the time being realize nothing of it.

How to Live, page 259

Animals are frequently killed that have been driven quite a distance to the slaughter. Their blood has become heated. They are of full flesh, and have been deprived of healthy exercise, and when they have to travel far, they become exhausted, and in that condition are killed for market. Their blood is highly inflamed, and those who eat of their meat, eat poison. Some are not immediately affected, while others are attacked with severe pain, and die from fever, cholera, or some unknown disease.... Some animals that are brought to the slaughter seem to realize what is to take place, and they become furious, and literally mad. They are killed while in this state, and their flesh is prepared for market. Their meat is poison, and has produced, in those who have eaten it, cramps, convulsions, apoplexy, and sudden death.

How to Live, page 59-60

Pulmonary diseases, cancers, and tumors are startlingly common among animals. It is true that the inspectors reject many cattle that are diseased, but many are passed on to the market that ought to have been refused.... Thus unwholesome flesh has gone on the market for human consumption. In many localities even fish is unwholesome, and ought not to be used. This is especially so where the fish come in contact with the sewerage of large cities.... The fish that partake of the filthy sewerage of the drains may pass into waters far distant from the sewerage, and be caught in localities where the water is pure and fresh; but because of the unwholesome drainage in which they have been feeding, they are not safe to eat.

Healthful Living, page 105

The fact that meat is largely diseased should lead us to make strenuous efforts to discontinue its use entirely.... It will be hard for some to do this, as hard as for the rum drinker to forsake his dram; but they will be better for the change.

Healthful Living, page 105

Water the Simplest of Remedies
Water is the best liquid possible to cleanse the tissues...drink some a little time before or after the meal.

Review and Herald, July 29, 1884

Eat sparingly, thus relieving the system of unnecessary burden, and encourage cheerfulness: take proper exercise in the open air, bathe frequently, and drink purely of pure, soft water.

Healthful Living, page 226

Water can be used in many ways to relieve suffering. Draughts of clear, hot water taken before eating (about half a quart, more or less), will never do any harm, but will rather be productive of good.

Letter 35, 1890

If they would become enlightened…and accustom themselves to outdoor exercise, and to air in their houses, summer and winter, and use soft water for drinking and bathing purposes, they would be comparatively well and happy, instead of dragging out a miserable existence.

How to Live, page 56

If, in their fevered state, water had been given them to drink freely, and applications had also been made externally, long days and nights of suffering would have been saved, and many precious lives spared.

How to Live, page 62

Many have never experienced the beneficial effects of water, and are afraid to use one of heaven's greatest blessings.

How to Live, page 62

Whether a person is sick or well, respiration is more free and easy if bathing is practiced. By it the muscles become more flexible, the body and mind are alike invigorated, and intellect is made brighter, and every faculty becomes livelier. The bath is a soother of the nerves. It promotes general perspiration, quickens the circulation, overcomes obstructions in the system, and acts beneficially on the kidneys and the urinary organs. Bathing helps the bowels, stomach, and liver, giving energy and new life to each. It also promotes digestion, and instead of the system's being weakened, it is strengthened. Instead of increasing the liability to cold, a bath, properly taken, fortifies against cold, because the circulation is improved, and the uterine organs, which are more or less congested, are relieved; for the blood is brought to the surface, and a more easy and regular flow of the blood through all of the blood vessels is obtained.

Testimonies for the Church, Volume 3, page 70

Nature, to relieve herself of poisonous impurities, makes an effort to free the system, which effort produces fevers and what is termed disease. But even then, if those who are afflicted, would assist nature in her efforts by the use of pure, soft water, much suffering would be prevented.

Selected Messages Book 2, page 460

It is not safe to trust to physicians who have not the fear of God before them. Without the influence of divine grace the hearts of men are "deceitful above all things, and desperately wicked." Self-aggrandizement is their aim. Under the cover of the medical profession what iniquities have been concealed, what delusions supported! The physician may claim to possess great wisdom and marvelous skill, when his character is abandoned and his practice contrary to the laws of life. The Lord our God assures us that He is waiting to be gracious; He invites us to call upon Him in the day of trouble. How can we turn from Him to trust in an arm of flesh.

Go with me to yonder sickroom. There lies a husband and father, a man who is a blessing to society and to the cause of God. He has been suddenly stricken down by disease. The fire of fever seems consuming him. He longs for pure water to moisten the parched lips, to quench the raging thirst, and cool the fevered brow. But, no; the doctor has forbidden water. The stimulus of strong drink is given and adds fuel to the fire. The blessed, heaven-sent water, skillfully applied, would quench the devouring flame; but it is set aside for poisonous drugs.

For a time nature wrestles for her rights; but at last, overcome, she gives up the contest, and death sets the sufferer free. God desired that man to live, to be a blessing to the world; Satan determined to destroy him, and through the agency of the physician he succeeded. How long shall we permit our most precious lights to be thus extinguished?

Testimonies, Vol. 5, pages 194, 195

Our sanitariums should be established in retired places that are free from all noise and confusion, such as the rumbling of carriages and streetcars.

The Lord his taught us that great efficacy for healing lies in a proper use of water. These treatments should be given skillfully. We have been instructed that in our treatment of the sick we should discard the use of drugs. There are simple herbs that can be used for the recovery of the sick, whose effect upon the system is very different from that of those drugs that poison the blood and endanger life.

Manuscript 73, 1908

Many have never experienced the beneficial effects of water, and are afraid to use one of Heaven's greatest blessings. Water has been refused persons suffering with burning fevers, through fear that it would injure them. If, in their fevered state, water had been given them to drink freely, and applications had also been made externally, long days and nights of suffering would have been saved, and many precious lives spared. But thousands have died with raging fevers consuming them, until the fuel which fed the fever was burnt up, the vitals consumed, and have died in the greatest agony, without being permitted to have water to allay their burning thirst. Water, which is allowed a senseless building, to put out the raging elements, is not allowed human beings to put out the fire which is consuming the vitals.

Spiritual Gifts, Vol.4, page 136-137

The things of nature are God's blessings, provided to give health to body, mind, and soul. They are given to the well to keep them well and to the sick to make them well. Connected with water treatment, they are more effective in restoring health than all the drug medication in the world.

Testimonies, Vol. 7, page 76

Exercise is Better Than Medicine

Inactivity is the greatest curse that could come upon most invalids. Light employment in useful labor, while it does not tax mind and body, has a happy influence upon both. It strengthens the muscles, improves the circulation, and gives the invalid the satisfaction of knowing that he is not wholly useless in this busy world. He may be able to do but little at first, but he will soon find his strength increasing and the amount of work done can be increased accordingly. Exercise aids the dyspeptic by giving the digestive organs a healthy tone...

Those whose habits are sedentary should, when the weather will permit, exercise in the open air every day, summer or winter. Walking is preferable to riding or driving, for it brings more of the muscles into exercise. The lungs are forced into healthy action, since it is impossible to walk briskly without inflating them. Such exercise would in many cases be better for the health than medicine.

Ministry of Healing, page 240
1905

Action is a law of our being. Every organ of the body has its appointed work, upon the performance of which its development and strength depend. The normal action of all the organs gives strength and vigor, while the tendency of disuse is toward decay and death. Bind up an arm, even for a few weeks, then free it from its bands, and you will see that it is weaker than the one you have been using moderately during the same time. Inactivity produces the same effect upon the whole muscular system.

Inactivity is a fruitful cause of disease. Exercise quickens and equalizes the circulation of the blood, but in idleness the blood does not circulate freely, and the changes in it, so necessary to life and health, do not take place. The skin, too, becomes inactive. Impurities are not expelled as they would be if the circulation had been quickened by vigorous exercise, the skin kept in a healthy condition, and the lungs fed with plenty of pure, fresh air.

This state of the system throws a double burden on the excretory organs, and disease is the result.

Ministry of Healing, pages 237-238

When invalids have nothing to occupy their time and attention, their thoughts become centered upon themselves, and they grow morbid and irritable. Many times they dwell upon their bad feelings until they think themselves much worse than they really are and wholly unable to do anything.

In all these cases well-directed physical exercise would prove an effective remedial agent. In some cases it is indispensable to the recovery of health. The will goes with the labor of the hands; and what these invalids need is to have the will aroused. When the will is dormant, the imagination becomes abnormal, and it is impossible to resist disease.

Notwithstanding all that is said and written concerning its importance, there are still many who neglect physical exercise. Some grow corpulent because the system is clogged; others become thin and feeble because their vital powers are exhausted in disposing of an excess of food. The liver is burdened in its effort to cleanse the blood of impurities, and illness is the result....

Such exercise would in many cases be better for the health than medicine. Physicians often advise their patients to take an ocean voyage, to go to some mineral spring, or to visit different places for change of climate, when in most cases if they would eat temperately, and take cheerful, healthful exercise, they would recover health and would save time and money.

Ministry of Healing, page 239-240

The Power of Pure, Fresh Air

In order to have good blood, we must breathe well. Full, deep inspirations of pure air, which fill the lungs with oxygen, purify the blood. They impart to it a bright color and send it, a life-giving current, to every part of the body. A good respiration soothes the nerves; it stimulates the appetite and renders digestion more perfect; and it induces sound, refreshing sleep."

Ministry of Healing, page 272

The lungs are constantly throwing off impurities, and they need to be constantly supplied with fresh air. Impure air does not afford the necessary supply of oxygen, and the blood passes to the brain and other organs without being vitalized. Hence the necessity of thorough ventilation. To live in close, ill-ventilated rooms, where the air is dead and vitiated, weakens the entire system. It becomes peculiarly sensitive to the influence of cold, and a slight exposure induces disease. It is close confinement indoors that makes many women pale and feeble. They breathe the same air over and over until it becomes laden with poisonous matter thrown off through the lungs and pores, and impurities are thus conveyed back to the blood.

Ministry of Healing, page 274

In the construction of buildings, whether for public purposes or as dwellings, care should be taken to provide for good ventilation and plenty of sunlight. Churches and schoolrooms are often faulty in this respect. Neglect of proper ventilation is responsible for much of the drowsiness and dullness that destroy the effect of many a sermon and make the teacher's work toilsome and ineffective.

Ministry of Healing, page 274

Many young children have passed five hours each day in schoolrooms not properly ventilated, nor sufficiently large for the healthful accommodation of the scholars. The air of such rooms soon becomes poison to the lungs that inhale it.

Testimonies for the Church, Vol. 3 page 135

Many families suffer with sore throat, lung diseases, and liver complaint, brought upon them by their own course of action. Their sleeping-rooms are small, unfit to sleep in for one night, but they occupy the small apartments for weeks, and months, and years.... They breathe the same air over and over, until it becomes impregnated with the poisonous impurities and waste matter thrown off from their bodies through the lungs and the pores of the skin.... Those who thus abuse their health must suffer with disease.

How to Live, page 63

Air, air, the precious boon of heaven, which all may have, will bless you with its invigorating influence if you will not refuse it entrance. Welcome it, cultivate a love for it, and it will prove a precious soother of the nerves.... The influence of pure, fresh air is to cause the blood to circulate healthfully through the system. It refreshes the body, and tends to render it strong and healthy, while at the same time its influence is decidedly felt upon the mind, imparting a degree of composure and serenity. It excites the appetite, and renders the digestion of food more perfect, and induces sound, sweet sleep.

Testimonies for the Church, Vol. 1 page 702

Sleeping-rooms especially should be well ventilated, and the atmosphere made healthy by light and air. Blinds should be left open several hours each day, the curtains put aside, and the room thoroughly aired.

Healthful Living, page 71

The studied habit of shunning the air and avoiding exercise closes the pores... making it impossible to throw off impurities through that channel. The burden of labor is thrown upon the liver, lungs, kidneys, etc., and these internal organs are compelled to do the work of the skin. Thus persons bring diseases upon themselves by their wrong habits.

Testimonies for the Church, Volume 2 page 524

Sunlight—A Great Healing Agent

If the windows were freed from blinds and heavy curtains, and the air in sun permitted to enter freely the darkened rooms, there would be seen a change for the better in the mental and physical health of the children. The pure air would have an invigorating influence upon them, and the sun that carries healing in its beams would soothe and cheer, and make them happy, joyous, and healthy.

The Health Reformer, April 1, 1871

Every room in our dwellings should be daily thrown open to the healthful rays of the sun, and the purifying air should be invited in. This will be a preventative of disease.

The Health Reformer, February 1, 1874

The feeble one should press out into the sunshine as earnestly and naturally as do the shaded plants and vines. The pale and sickly grain blade that has struggled up out of the cold of early spring, puts out the natural and healthy deep green after enjoying for a few days the health-and-life-giving rays of the sun. Go out into the light and warmth of the glorious sun, you pale and sickly ones, and share with vegetation its life-giving, health-dealing power.

The Health Reformer, May 1, 1871

The Power of Roots and Herbs

I have always used red clover top, as I stated to you. I offered you this, and told you it was a good, simple, and wholesome drink.

Letter 12, 1888

The Lord has given some simple herbs of the field that at times are beneficial; and if every family understood how to use these herbs in case of sickness, much suffering might be prevented and no doctor need be called. These old-fashioned, simple herbs, used intelligently, would have recovered many sick who have died under drug medication.

Manuscript 162, 1897

This is God's method. The herbs that grow for the benefit of man, and the little handful of herbs kept and steeped and used for sudden ailments, have served tenfold, yes, one hundred fold better purposes, than all the drugs hidden under mysterious names and dealt out to the sick.

The Paulson Collection of Ellen G. White Letters. page 31

There are herbs that are harmless, the use of which will tide over many apparently serious difficulties. But if all would seek to become intelligent in regard to their bodily necessities, sickness would be rare instead of common. An ounce of prevention is worth a pound of cure.

Manuscript 86, 1897

Christ never planted the seeds of death in the system. Satan planted these seeds when he tempted Adam to eat of the tree of knowledge, which meant disobedience to God. Not one noxious plant was placed in the Lord's great garden, but after Adam and Eve sinned, poisonous herbs sprang up. In the parable of the sower the question was asked the Master, "Didst not thou sow good seed in thy field? How then hath it tares?" The master answered, "An enemy hath done this." All tares are sown by the evil one. Every noxious herb is of his sowing, and by his ingenious

90

methods of amalgamation he has corrupted the earth with tares. Then shall physicians continue to resort to drugs which leave a deadly evil in the system, destroying that life which Christ came to restore? Christ's remedies cleanse the system. But Satan has tempted man to introduce into the system that which weakens the human machinery, clogging and destroying the fine, beautiful arrangements of God. The drugs administered to the sick do not restore, but destroy. Drugs never cure. Instead, they place in the system seeds which bear a very bitter harvest....

Our Savior is the restorer of the moral image of God in man. He has supplied in the natural world remedies for the ills of man, that His followers may have life and that they may have it more abundantly. We can with safety discard the concoctions which man has used in the past. The Lord has provided antidotes for disease in simple plants, and these can be used by faith, with no denial of faith; for by using the blessings provided by God for our benefit we are cooperating with Him. He can use water and sunshine and the herbs which He has caused to grow in healing maladies brought on by indiscretion or accident. We do not manifest a lack of faith when we ask God to bless His remedies. True faith will thank God for the knowledge of how to use these precious blessings in a way which will restore mental and physical vigor.

Manuscript 65, 1899

A cup of tea made from catnip herb will quiet the nerves. Hop tea will induce sleep. Hop poultices over the stomach will relieve pain. If eyes are weak, if there is pain in the eyes, or inflammation, soft flannel cloths wet in hot water and salt, will bring relief quickly.

When the head is congested, if the feet and limbs are put in a bath with a little mustard, relief will be obtained.

If the eyes are weak, if there is pain in the eyes, or inflammation, soft flannel cloths wet in hot water and salt, will bring relief quickly.

The Place of Herbs in Rational Therapy, page 6

There are many more simple remedies, which will do much to restore healthful action to the body. All these simple preparations the Lord expects us to use for ourselves; but man's extremities are God's opportunities.

If we neglect to do that which is within the reach of nearly every family, and ask the Lord to relieve pain, when we are too indolent to make use of these remedies within our power, it is simply presumption. The Lord expects us to work in order that we may obtain food. He does not propose that we shall gather the harvest unless we break the sod, till the soil, and cultivate the produce. Then God sends the rain and the sunshine and the clouds to cause vegetation to flourish. God works, and man cooperates with God. Then there is seed time and harvest.

Letter 35, 1890

It is not a denial of faith to use such remedies as God has provided to alleviate pain and to aid nature in her work of restoration...We should employ every facility for the restoration of health, taking every advantage possible, working in harmony with natural laws.

Ministry of Healing, page 231-232

The simpler remedies are less harmful (than drug poisons) in proportion to their simplicity, but in very many cases these are used when not at all necessary.

The Place of Herbs in Rational Therapy, page 8

If we neglect to do that which is within the reach of nearly every family, and ask the Lord to relieve pain, when we are too indolent to make use of these remedies within our power, it is simply presumption. The Lord expects us to work in order that we may obtain food. He does not propose we shall gather the harvest unless we break the sod, till the soil, and cultivate the produce. Then God sends the rain and the sunshine and the clouds to cause vegetation to flourish. God works and man cooperates with God. Then there is seedtime and harvest. God has caused to grow out of the ground herbs for the use of man, and if we understand the nature of these roots and herbs, and make a right use of them, there would not be a necessity of running for the doctor so frequently, and people would be in much better health than they are today.

Medical Ministry, pages. 230- 231

The intricate names given the medicines are used to cover up the matter, so that none will know what is given them as remedies unless they obtain a dictionary to find out the meaning of these names. The Lord has given some simple herbs of the field that at times are beneficial; and if every family were educated in how to use these herbs in case of sickness, much suffering might be prevented, and no doctor need be called. These old-fashioned, simple herbs, used intelligently, would have recovered many sick, who have died under drug medication.

Letter 82, 1897

The Healing Value of Charcoal

One of the most beneficial remedies is pulverized charcoal, placed in a bag and used in fomentations. This is a most successful remedy. If wet in smartweed boiled, it is still better. I have ordered this in cases where the sick were suffering great pain, and when it has been confided to me by the physician that he thought it was the last before the close of life.

Then I suggested the charcoal, and the patient slept, the turning point came, and recovery was the result. To students when injured with bruised hands and suffering with inflammation, I have prescribed this simple remedy, with perfect success. The poison of inflammation was overcome, the pain removed, and healing went on rapidly. The most severe inflammation of the eyes will be relieved by a poultice of charcoal, put in a bag, and dipped in hot or cold water, as will best suit the case. This works like a charm.

I expect you will laugh at this, but if I could give this remedy some outlandish name, that no one knew but myself, it would have greater influence. But Dr. Kellogg, many things have been opened before me that no one but myself is any the wiser for in regard to the management of sickness and disease,—the effect of the use of drug medication, the thousands in our work who might have lived if they had not sent for a physician, and had let nature work the recovery herself. But the simplest remedies may assist nature, and leave no baleful effects after their use.

Letter 82, 1897

On one occasion a physician came to me in great distress. He had been called to attend a young woman who was dangerously ill. She had contracted fever while on the campground and was taken to our school building, near Melbourne, Australia. But she became so much worse that it was feared she could not live.

The physician, Dr. Merritt Kellogg, came to me and said, "Sister White, have you any light for me on this case? If relief cannot be given our sister, she can live but a few hours." I replied, "Send to a blacksmith's shop and get some pulverized charcoal; make a poultice of it, and lay it over her stomach and sides." The doctor hastened away to follow out my instructions. Soon he returned, saying, "Relief came in less than half an hour after the application of the poultices. She is now having the first natural sleep she has had for days."

I have ordered the same treatment for others who were suffering great pain, and it has brought relief, and been the means of saving life. My mother had told me that snake bites and the sting of reptiles and poisonous insects could often be rendered harmless by the use of charcoal poultices. When working on the land at Avondale, Australia, the workmen would often bruise their hands and limbs, and this in many cases resulted in such severe inflammation that the worker would have to leave his work for some time.

One came to me one day in this condition, with his hand tied in a sling. He was much troubled over the circumstances; for his help was needed in clearing the land. I said to him, "Go to the place where you have been burning the timber, and get me some charcoal from the eucalyptus tree, and pulverize it, and I will dress your hand." This was done, and the next morning he reported that the pain was gone. Soon he was ready to return to his work.

I write these things that you may know that the Lord has not left us without the use of simple remedies which when used will not leave the system in the weakened condition in which the use of drugs so often leaves it. We need well trained nurses who can understand how to use the simple remedies that nature provides for restoration to health, and who can teach those who are ignorant of the laws of health how to use these simple but effective cures.

Letter 90, 1908

I will tell you a little about my experience which charcoal as a remedy. For some forms of indigestion, it is more efficacious than drugs. A little olive oil into which some of this powder has been stirred tends to cleanse and heal. I find it is excellent...

Always study and teach the use of the simplest remedies, and the special blessing of the Lord may be expected to follow the use of these means which are within the reach of the common people.

Letter 100, 1903

Medicinal Properties of the Trees

In a certain place, preparations were being made to clear the land for the erection of a sanitarium. Light was given that there is health in the fragrance of the pine, the cedar, and the fir. And there are several other kinds of trees that have medicinal properties that are health-promoting. Let not such trees be ruthlessly cut down. Better change the site of the building than cut down these evergreen trees.

Letter 95, 1902

I have already told you the remedy I use when suffering from difficulties with my throat. I take a glass of boiled honey, and into this I put a few drops of eucalyptus oil, stirring it in well. When the cough comes on, I take a teaspoonful of this mixture, and relief comes almost immediately. I have always used this with the best results. I ask you to use the same remedy when you are troubled with the cough. This prescription may seem so simple that you feel no confidence in it, but I have tried it for a number of years, and can highly recommend it.

Letter 20, 1909

I have had considerable trouble with my throat, but whenever I use this [eucalyptus and honey], I overcome the difficulty very quickly. I have to use it only a few times, and the cough is removed. If you will use this prescription, you may be your own physician. If the first trial does not effect a cure, try it again. The best time to take it is before retiring.

Letter 348, 1908

Take warm footbaths, into which have been put the leaves from the eucalyptus tree. There is great virtue in these leaves, and if you will try this, you will prove my words to be true. The oil of the eucalyptus is especially beneficial in case of cough and pains in the chest and lungs. I want you to make a trial of this remedy which is so simple, and which costs you nothing.

Letter 20, 1909

Helping Others: A Cure for Disease

You who are suffering with poor health, there is a remedy for you. If you clothe the naked, and bring the poor that are cast out to thy house, and deal thy bread to the hungry, "then shall thy light break forth as the morning, and thine health shall spring forth speedily." Doing good is an excellent remedy for disease.

Testimonies for the Church, Volume 2, page 29

The consciousness of right-doing is the best medicine for diseased bodies and minds. He who is at peace with God has secured the most important requisite to health. The blessing of the Lord is life to the receiver.

Signs of the Times, June 15, 1882

Doing good is a work that benefits both giver and receiver. If you forget self in your interest for others, you gain a victory over your infirmities. The satisfaction you will realize in doing good will aid you greatly in the recovery of the healthy tone of the imagination. The pleasure of doing good animates the mind and vibrates through the whole body.

Testimonies for the Church, Volume 2, page 534

Sickness of the mind prevails everywhere. Nine tenths of the diseases from which men suffer have their foundation here...The religion of Christ, so far from being the cause of insanity, is one of its most effectual remedies: for it is a potent soother of the nerves.

Testimonies for the Church, Volume 5, page 443

A person whose mind is quiet and satisfied in God is in the pathway to health.

Review and Herald, March 11, 1880

A sore, sick heart, a discouraged mind, needs mild treatment: and it is through tender sympathy that this class of minds can be healed. The physician should first gain their confidence, and then point them to the all-healing Physician. If their minds can be directed to the Burden-Bearer, and they can have faith that He will have an interest in them, the cure of their diseased bodies and minds will be sure.

Testimonies for the Church, Volume 3, page 184

In every large city there should be a representation of true medical missionary work. Let many now ask: "Lord, what wilt Thou have me to do?" Acts 9:6. It is the Lord's purpose that His method of healing without drugs shall be brought into prominence in every large city through our medical institutions. God invests with holy dignity those who go forth farther and still farther, in every place to which it is possible to obtain entrance.

Testimonies, vol. 9, page 169

The ambassadors of Christ can be doubly useful if they know how to restore the diseased to health. This was the work of Christ. But as in prayer we present these suffering ones to the Lord for His healing power to come to them, the people themselves must be instructed to do those things which will assist nature, not in drug medication, but in the use of the agencies the Lord has prepared,—sunlight, pure air, pure water, healthful exercise. These things possess a power which millions in our world know nothing of. These restoring agencies must be used intelligently, and as we do all that it is in our power to do, we must mingle with our work our earnest prayers.

Manuscript 110, 1898

Thousands need and would gladly receive instruction concerning the simple methods of treating the sick—methods that are taking the place of the use of poisonous drugs. There is great need of instruction in regard to dietetic reform. Wrong habits of eating and the use of unhealthful food are in no small degree responsible for the intemperance and crime and wretchedness that curse the world.

Ministry of Healing, page 146

Trust in Divine Power

While the Physician uses nature's remedies for physical disease, he should point his patients to Him who can relieve the maladies of both the soul and the body.

Ministry of Healing, page 111

The physician needs more than human wisdom and power that he may know how to minister to the many perplexing cases of disease of the mind and heart with which he is called to deal. If he is ignorant of the power of divine grace, he cannot help the afflicted one, but will aggravate the difficulty; but if he has a firm hold upon God, he will be able to help the diseased, distracted mind.

Testimonies for the Church, Vol. 5, page 444

The physician should educate the people to look from the human to the Divine. Instead of teaching the sick to depend upon human beings for the cure of soul and body, he should direct them to the One who can save to the uttermost all who come unto Him. He who made man's mind knows what the mind needs. God alone is the One who can heal. Those whose minds and bodies are diseased are to behold in Christ the restorer. "Because I live," He says, "ye shall live also." John 14:19. This is the life we are to present to the sick, telling them that if they have faith in Christ as the restorer, if they co-operate with Him, obeying the laws of health, and striving to perfect holiness in His fear, He will impart to them His life. When we present to them Christ in this way, we are imparting a power, a strength, that is of value; for it comes from above. This is the true science of healing for body and soul!

Counsels on Health, page 386

No one ever trusted God in vain. He will never disappoint those who put their trust in Him.

Testimonies for the Church, Vol. 9, page 213

"The Savior would have us encourage the sick, the hopeless, the afflicted, to take hold upon His strength.

Through faith and prayer the sickroom may be transformed into a Bethel. In word and deed, physicians and nurses may say, so plainly that it cannot be misunderstood, "God is in this place" to save, and not to destroy. Christ desire to manifest His presence in the sickroom, filling the hearts of physicians and nurses with the sweetness of His love. If the life of the attendants upon the sick is such that Christ can go with them to the bedside of the patient, there will come to him the conviction that the compassionate Savior is present; and this conviction will itself do much for the healing o of both the soul and the body." EGW

Ministry of Healing, page 232

To talk of religion in a casual way, to pray without soul hunger and living faith, avails nothing. A nominal faith in Christ, which accepts Him merely as the Saviour of the world, can never bring healing to the soul. The faith that is unto salvation is not a mere intellectual assent to the truth. He who waits for entire knowledge before he will exercise faith cannot receive blessing from God. It is not enough to believe about Christ; we must believe IN Him. The only faith that will benefit us is that which embraces Him as a personal Saviour; which appropriates His merits to ourselves. Many hold faith as an opinion. Saving faith is a transaction by which those who receive Christ join themselves in covenant relation with God. Genuine faith is life. A living faith means an increase of vigor, a confiding trust, by which the soul becomes a conquering power."

The Desire of Ages, page 347

Other Miscellaneous Remedies

Grape Juice and Eggs: I have told you what I have because I have received light that you are injuring your body by a poverty-stricken diet. I must say to you that it will not be best for you to instruct the students as you have done in regard to the diet question, because your ideas in regard to discarding certain things will not be for the help of those who need help...It is a lack of suitable food that has cause you to suffer so keenly. You have not taken the food essential to nourish your frail physical strength.

You must not deny yourself of good wholesome food...Get eggs of healthy fowls. Use these eggs cooked or raw. Drop them uncooked into the best unfermented wine you can find. This will supply that which is necessary to your system.

Counsels on Diet and Foods, pages 203-204

Blood Transfusions: There is one thing that has saved life,—an infusion of blood from one person to another; but this would be difficult and perhaps impossible for you to do. I merely suggest it.

Letter 37, 1901

Figs for Hezekiah: When the Lord told Hezekiah that He would spare his life for fifteen years, and as a sign that He would fulfill His promise, caused the sun to go back ten degrees. Why did He not put His direct, restoring power upon the King? He told him to apply a bunch of figs to his sore, and that natural remedy, blessed by God, healed him.

The God of nature directs the human agent to use natural remedies now.

Letter 182, 1899

Powder for Cancer Sufferers: I have just received a letter from Brother Stephen Belden of Norfolk Island. He is afflicted with a cancer. Brother Alfred Nobbs, the elder of the Norfolk Island Church, has also been afflicted with what appeared to be a cancer. He went to Sydney, and his face and head were badly cut in removing the cancer. But he received little help, and he still continues to suffer greatly.

Brother Stephen Belden has a cancer on his ear. I thought that if you would send him powders at once, with directions for their use, Brother Belden and Brother Nobbs might both be benefited by their use.

Will you kindly respond by sending the powders as soon as you receive this letter?

I am not well today, so cannot write much. I will send you this line, hoping that you will send the powders.

Letter 236, 1906

Note: *The value of this communication lies, not in the power Dr. Gibbs might suggest which might bring relief in the cancer case, but in the fact that Mrs. White was eager to have use made of a powder she hoped might be a remedy. A. L. White*

Specific Counsel to Doctors

Reform and Humility Needed

In regard to hygienic methods and the disuse of drugs, from the light God has given me, there must be a reform. Our people are going far from the light which God has given on this subject. If Dr. B or Dr. A or any other doctor goes into the institution, he must work in harmony with the light God has seen fit to give to His people in reform methods of treatment. If Dr. and his wife unite with Dr. B or any other physician, all egotism must be done away. The spirit that controlled the medical fraternity has been of that character which will exclude many from heaven unless they put away this spirit and work with the mind and spirit of Christ. Wicked jealousies, evil thinking, evil speaking of their brethren, has been an offence to God. The methods of drug medication have created the bitterest animosity in feeling, almost equal to the prejudice that Catholics have manifested toward Protestants because they did not view every point of religious faith as they themselves.

Such a spirit may be expected in the world, but when it becomes a controlling power among Christians, it is an offence to God. It is a shame when manifested among those who profess to be followers of Jesus. There must be a reform among the medical fraternity or the church will be purged from those who will not be Bible Christians. It is altogether too late in the day for such a Satanic exhibition of spirit as is revealed among medical drug practitioners.

God abhors it. I could write much on this subject, but I am not able now.

Letter 48, 1892

I wish I could see you face to face, but as I cannot, I will write. Thank you for your prescription. I will be careful. The Lord help me, is my prayer, and I pray that the Lord may help you, my brother, that you may not take on too many burdens, and by so doing disqualify yourself for the management of them...

The influence you have gained in the medical profession is large and broad, and in some respects it has been as God would have it. You have caused the light God has given you to shine forth to others, and this light has influenced others to labor in the different lines in the medical work. But according to the light the Lord has given me, something of the spirit of Free Masonry exists, and has built a wall about the work. The old regular practice has been exalted as the only true method for the treatment of disease. And to a large degree this feeling has leavened the physicians connected with you. They have resorted to drugs in cases of fever to break it up, as they have thought. This method has broken up fevers and other diseases, but it has in some cases broken up the whole man with it.

The Lord has been pleased to present this matter before me in clear lines. Fever cases need not be treated with drugs. The most difficult cases are best and most successfully managed by nature's own resources. This science, fully adopted, will bring the best results, if the practitioner will be thorough. The Lord will bless the physician who depends on natural methods, helping every function of the human machinery to act in its own strength the part the Lord designed it to act in restoring itself to proper action.

Dr. Kellogg, God has given you favor with the medical fraternity, and He would have you hold that favor. But in no case are you to stand as do the physicians of the world to exalt Allopathy above every other practice, and call all other methods quackery and error; for from the beginning to the present time the results of Allopathy have made a most objectionable showing. There has been loss of life in your sanitarium because drugs have been administered, and these give no chance for nature to do her work of restoration. Drug medication has broken up the power of the human machinery, and the patients have died. Others have carried the drugs away with them, making less effective the simple remedies nature uses to restore the system. The students in your institution are not to be educated to regard drugs as a necessity. They are to be educated to leave drugs alone.

The medical fraternity, represented to me as Free Masonry, with their long, unintelligible names, which common people cannot understand, would call the Lord's prescription for Hezekiah quackery. Death was pronounced upon the king, but he prayed for life, and his prayer was heard. Those who had the care of him were told to get a bunch of figs and put them on the sore, and the king was restored. This means was taken by God to teach them that all their preparations were only depriving the king of the power to rally and overcome disease. While they pursued their course of treatment, his life could not be saved. The Lord diverted their minds from their wonderful mysteries to a simple remedy of nature. There are lessons for us all in these directions. Young men who are sent to Ann Arbor to obtain an education which they think will exalt them as supreme in their treatment of disease by drugs, will find that it will result in the loss of life rather than restoration to health and strength. These mixtures place a double taxation upon nature, and in the effort to throw off the poisons they contain, thousands of persons lose their lives. We must leave drugs entirely alone, for in using them we introduce an enemy into the system. I write this because we have to meet this drug medication in the physicians in this country, and we do not want this practice as in Battle Creek to steal into our midst as a thief. We want the door closed against the enemy before the lives of human beings are imperiled.

Letter 67, 1899

It would have been better if those sent from our schools to Ann Arbor had never had any connection with that institution. The education in drug medication and the false religious theories have brought forth a class of practitioners who need to unlearn much they have learned. They need to obtain an altogether different experience before they can say in word and indeed, We are medical missionaries. Till they obtain such an experience, the great Physician does not acknowledge them as medical missionaries. They come on to the platform of action unprepared for the high and holy work which needs to be done at this time.

Letter 3, 1901

There is to be a sanitarium in Australia, and altogether new methods of treating the sick are to be practiced. Drug medication must be left out of the question, if the human physician would receive the diploma written and issued in heaven. There are many physicians who will never receive this diploma unless they learn in the school of the great Physician. This means that they must unlearn and cast away the supposed wonderful knowledge of how to treat disease with poisonous drugs. The must go to God's great laboratory of nature, and there learn the simplest methods of using the remedies which the Lord has furnished. When drugs are thrown aside, when fermented liquor of all kinds is discarded, when God's remedies, sunshine, pure air, water, and good food are used, there will be far fewer deaths and a far greater number of cures.

Manuscript 65
1899

The students at Loma Linda are seeking for an education that is after the Lord's order, an education that will help them to develop into successful teachers and laborers for others. When their education at Loma Linda is completed, they should be able to go forth and join the intelligent workers in the world's great harvest fields who are carrying forward the work of reform that is to prepare a people to stand in the day of Christ's coming. Everywhere workers are needed to know how to combat disease and give skillful care to the sick and suffering. We should do all in our power to enable those who desire to be thus fitted for service to gain the necessary training...

Our people should become intelligent in the treatment of sickness without the aid of poisonous drugs. Many should seek to obtain the education that will enable them to combat disease in its various forms by the most simple methods. Thousands have gone down to the grave because of the use of poisonous drugs, who might have been restored to health by simple methods of treatment. Water treatments, wisely and skillfully given, may be the means of saving many lives. Let diligent study be united with careful treatments. Let prayers of faith be offered by the bedside of the sick. Let the sick be encouraged to claim the promises of God for themselves.

Medical Ministry, pages 56-57

Let the students be given a practical education. The less dependent you are upon worldly methods of education, the better it will be for the students. Special instruction should be given in the art of training the sick without the use of poisonous drugs and in harmony with the light that God has given. In the treatment of the sick, poisonous drugs need not be used. Students should come forth from the school without having sacrificed the principles of health reform or their love for God and righteousness.

The education that meets the world's standard is to be less and less valued by those who are seeking for efficiency in carrying the medical missionary work in connection with the work of the third angel's message. They are to be educated from the standpoint of conscience, and, as they conscientiously and faithfully follow right methods in their treatment of the sick, these methods will come to be recognized and preferable to the methods to which many have become accustomed, which demand the use of poisonous drugs.

We should not at this time seek to compete with worldly medical schools. Should we do this, our chances of success would be small.

Testimonies, Vol. 9, pages 175-176

The Lord calls for the best talents to be united at this center [Loma Linda] for the carrying on of the work as He has directed,—not the talent that will demand the largest salary, but the talent that will place itself on the side of Christ to work in His lines. We must have medical instructors who will teach the science of healing without the use of drugs...We are to prepare a company of workers who will follow Christ's methods.

Medical Ministry, page 75

Let the instruction be given in simple words. We have no need to use the many expressions used by worldly physicians which are so difficult to understand that they must be interpreted by the physician. These long names are often used to conceal the character of the drugs being used to combat disease. We do not need these. Nature's simple remedies will aid in recovery without leaving the deadly after-effects so often felt by those who use poisonous drugs.

Letter 82, 1908

The work of the physician must begin in an understanding of the works and teachings of the Great Physician. Christ left the courts of heaven that He might minister to the sick and suffering of earth. We must cooperate with the Chief of physicians, walking in all humility of mind before Him. Then the Lord will bless our earnest efforts to relieve suffering humanity. It is not by the use of poisonous drugs that this will be done, but by the use of simple remedies. We should seek to correct false habits and practices, and teach the lessons of self-denial. The indulgence of appetite is the greatest evil with which we have to contend.

Medical Ministry, page 85

I found an article that I had written about a year ago, in reference to the establishment of a school of the highest order, in which the students would not be taught to use drugs in the treatment of the sick.

Letter 360

Those who desire to become missionaries are to hear instruction from competent physicians, who will teach them how to care for the sick without the use of drugs. Such lessons will be of the highest value to those who go out to labor in foreign countries. And the simple remedies used will save many lives.

Medical Ministry, page 231

It is not necessary that our medical missionaries follow the precise track marked out by medical men of the world. They do not need to administer drugs to the sick. They do not need to follow the drug medication in order to have influence in their work.

The message was given me that if they would consecrate themselves to the Lord, if they would seek to obtain under men ordained of God a thorough knowledge of their work, the Lord would make them skillful.

Some of our medical missionaries have supposed that a medical training according to the plans of worldly schools is essential to their success.

To those who have thought that the only way to success is by being taught by worldly men and by pursuing a course that is sanctioned by worldly men, I would now say, "Put away such ideas. This is a mistake that should be corrected. It is a dangerous thing to catch the spirit of the world; the popularity which such a course invites, will bring into the work a spirit which the Word of God cannot sanction."

It is a lack of faith in the power of God that leads our physicians to lean so much on the arm of the law, and to trust so much to the influence of worldly powers. The true medical missionary will be wise in the treatment of the sick, using the remedies that nature provides.

And then he will look to Christ as the true healer of diseases. The principles of health reform brought into the life of the patient, the use of nature's remedies, and the cooperation of divine agencies in behalf of the suffering, will bring success.

I am instructed to say that in our educational work there is to be no compromise in order to meet the world's standards. God's commandment-keeping people are not to unite with the world to carry various lines of work according to worldly plans and worldly wisdom...

Facilities should be provided at Loma Linda, that the necessary instruction in medical lines may be given by instructors who fear the Lord, and who are in harmony with His plans for the treatment of the sick.

Review and Herald
March 6, 1913

The Lord has connected Dr. Kellogg with the medical fraternity outside our people. His influence has had much to do with the abolishing of drugs to a large extent, and the introduction of nature's own restoratives. This work has not been done by making a raid upon drugs, for it needed the wisdom of a serpent and the harmlessness of a dove. Dr. Kellogg's connection with God enables him to take the presence of the Holy Spirit with him into assemblies where there is generally much levity, and where many things are spoken that might better be left unsaid. The people respect the doctor's religious principles, and show that they are somewhat under the influence of this faith.

Letter 38, 1899

As to drugs being used in our institutions, it is contrary to the light which the Lord has been pleased to give. The drugging business has done more harm to our world and killed more than it has helped or cured. The light was first given to me why institutions should be established, that is, sanitariums were to reform the medical practices of physicians.

Medical Ministry, page 27

Doctors Held Accountable by God

There is a terrible account to be rendered to God by men who have so little regard for human life as to treat the body so ruthlessly in dealing out their drugs. It is the duty of every person to become intelligent in regard to disease and its cause. We must study our Bible in order to understand the value that the Lord places upon the men and women whom Christ has purchased at purchased at such an infinite price. Then we should become acquainted with the laws of life, that every action of the human agent may be in perfect harmony with the laws of God. When there is so great peril in ignorance, is it not best to be wise in regard to the human habitation, fitted up by our Creator, and over which He desires we shall be faithful stewards? We are not excusable if through ignorance we destroy God's building by taking into our stomachs poisonous drugs under a variety of names we do not understand. It is our duty to refuse all such prescriptions.

Manuscript 44, 1896

This is a matter of grave responsibility. God holds men and women accountable to keep themselves in the very best health, physically, mentally, and morally, that they may distinguish between the sacred and the common. The laws which God has established for the well-being of the physical structure are to be treated as divine. To every action done in violation of these laws a penalty is affixed. The transgressor is recorded as having broken the commandments of God.

Many seem to think that it is their privilege to treat their bodies as they please. Do such stop to consider that God requires them to obey His physical laws, and that for their violation of these laws they must answer at His bar?

Manuscript 155, 1899
Temperance from a Christian Standpoint

Correspondence with a Medical Student

A young medical student, Edgar Caro, once wrote Ellen White for more specific answers regarding the use of prescription medications in medical practice. His letter and her answer, which may be helpful to all of us, are included below?

The Letter

Hearing so much about you from my dear mother, and knowing how interested you are in the medical branch of our work, and how much God has revealed to you concerning this, I have decided to take a little of your time to ask a question which has troubled several of our medical students.

Next year a good number of us enter upon our last and most important year of the medical course at the university. From our study of the *Testimonies* and the little work, *How to Live*, we can see that the Lord is strongly opposed to the use of drugs in our medical work.

We believed they were harmful because the Lord has said so through the *Testimonies*. Now we know from our three years' study that 'drugging' is a most unscientific practice.

Several of the students are in doubt as to the meaning of the word 'drug' as mentioned in *How to Live*. Does it refer only to the stronger medicines as mercury, strychnine, arsenic, and such poisons, the things we medical students call 'drugs,' or does it also include the simple remedies, as potassium, iodine, squills, etc. We know that our success will be proportionate to our adherence to God's methods. For this reason I have asked the above question.

From Letter Written by Edgar Caro
to Mrs. E.G. White, Aug. 15, 1893

Ellen White's Answer

Your questions, I will say, are answered largely, if not definitely, in How to Live. Drug poisons mean the articles which you have mentioned. The simpler remedies are less harmful in proportion to their simplicity; but in very many cases these are used when not at all necessary. There are simple herbs and roots that every family may use for themselves, and need not call a physician any sooner than they would call a lawyer. I do not think that I can give you any definite line of medicines compounded and dealt out by doctors, that are perfectly harmless. And yet it would not be wisdom to engage in controversy over this subject.

The practitioners are very much in earnest in using their dangerous concoctions, and I am decidedly opposed to resorting to such things. They never cure; they may change the difficulty to create a worse one. Many of those who practice the prescribing of drugs, would not take the same or give them to their children. If they have an intelligent knowledge of the human body, if they understand the delicate, wonderful human machinery, they must know that we are fearfully and wonderfully made, and that not a particle of these strong drugs should be introduced into this human living organism.

As the matter was laid open before me, and the sad burden of the result of drug medication, the light was given me so that Seventh-day Adventists should establish health institutions, discarding all these health-destroying inventions, and physicians should treat the sick upon hygienic principles. The great burden should be to have well-trained nurses, and well-trained medical practitioners to educate "precept upon precept; line upon line, line upon line; here a little, and there a little."

Train the people to correct habits and healthful practices, remembering that an ounce of prevention is of more value than a pound of cure. Lectures and studies in this line will prove of the highest value...

Letter 17-a, 1893
Answer to Edgar Caro, Napier, New Zealand
Oct. 2, 1893

Made in United States
North Haven, CT
11 January 2024

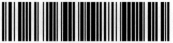

47316857R00067